THE
COMPLETE
PROSTATE
HANDBOOK

Anne Charlish

THE COMPLETE PROSTATE HANDBOOK

*Published in Great Britain MCMXCVI by Carnell plc,
28 Eccleston Square, London SW1V 1PU*

Copyright © MCMXCVI by Carnell plc.

Typeset by Typesetting Solutions, Slough, Berks.

Printed by Repro City Limited, London.

ISBN 1-85779-887-2

Table of Contents

The foreword that follows has been provided by Dr Steve Carroll, MB, BS, MRCS, LRCP.

Dr Carroll is a former GP and is now Director of a leading international health care public relations agency. He has written on medical and health issues for both consumer and professional publications. Health education is his speciality. He is author of *The Complete Family Guide to Healthy Living* and *The Which? Guide to Men's Health,* and has contributed to many other health books as well as writing regularly for several magazines. Dr Carroll's other main interest is sports medicine. He was previously Assistant Team Doctor for Tottenham Hotspur Football Club and Expedition Doctor for the Ian Botham Hannibal Charity Trek across the Alps.

Foreword

Men visit their doctors much less frequently than women, not because women suffer from more illnesses than men but because women are much more knowledgeable and concerned about their own health. A recent MORI poll, conducted in July 1992, showed that a large proportion of men – around 21 per cent –were either reluctant to go to their doctor, or needed encouragement to do so. Men are not only badly informed about their health, they would actually rather not know. The same MORI poll showed that only 32 per cent of men know anything about their prostate gland. Yet the figures on prostate disease are well-established, showing that prostate disease causes four times the number of deaths resulting from cervical cancer, and that more than one man in three is likely to suffer from some form of prostate disease before the age of 50.

Men tend, too, to lead much less healthy lifestyles than women. They are more likely to drink too much alcohol, to smoke, to eat badly, to take too little exercise, and to deal less than efficiently with stress.

It is true that some men nowadays are beginning to take a greater interest in their health and to adopt a healthier outlook. But this applies only to a small minority of men.

It's their body, their life, and it will serve them well if they look after it and keep a wary eye on what can go wrong with it. I hope that this book will be read not only be concerned female partners but by men themselves. After all, it is them that it concerns. Reading it will not guarantee them a long life, totally free from prostate disease. But it will give them a better chance of taking control of those factors that may affect the health of their prostate and of dealing with things should they go wrong.

Taking responsibility for their health is one of the most important things that men can do. It will give them a new sense of worth and it will, in the process, give them a better quality of life.

Dr Steve Carroll
London
1996

1 Introduction

ALL MALES ARE BORN with a prostate gland and, as with many other organs in the body, they will be happily unaware of its presence unless it causes problems. About the size of a chestnut in the adult male, the prostate gland encircles the outlet of the bladder, which is called the urethra.

Unfortunately, as men grow older the prostate gland is a common source of discomfort, often causing acute problems to the sufferer, as well as having a serious impact on their quality of life. According to a survey by the World Health Organisation, as many as 80 per cent of men are likely to experience prostate problems at some point in their lives, which indicates that knowledge of this organ is vital to the majority of men.

The purpose of this book is to increase awareness of the prostate gland and the problems which can arise. Firstly, the book explains the nature and functions of the prostate gland, and then goes on to discuss what can go wrong, the diagnosis of problems, and probably most importantly for the sufferer, the various treatments which can be employed to alleviate or cure the symptoms. Finally, there is a section on commonly asked questions, together with answers.

It is hoped that the information within this book will serve to enlighten men about the prostate gland and what can go wrong, giving them the confidence to seek early advice and not assume that their problems are due to 'their age' and that 'nothing can be done'. This is not so. Many positive advances in treatment are being made and will be described in the forthcoming chapters.

WHAT IS THE PROSTATE GLAND?

The prostate gland is a tiny part of the male body, about the size of a chestnut, yet it can cause a disproportionately large number of problems. The great majority of these problems are irritating and inconvenient, and can have a dramatic effect on lifestyle rather than in any way life-threatening, though some of them can be very serious indeed.

The prostate is not just one gland. It is, in fact, a complex gland, consisting of millions of tiny glands, lined with cells that secrete fluids, which empty into tens of thousands of tubules and ducts, and eventually into the urethra through 14-18 exits.

The prostate gland is involved in the reproductive process, in that prostate secretions in semen are important providers of nutrients for sperm. The prostate gland is known as an accessory sex gland, in that it is made up of glandular tissue and plays only a secondary role in the reproductive process.

PROSTATE PROBLEMS

According to the World Health Organization (WHO), as many as 80 per cent of men are likely to experience prostate problems at some point in their lives. Many of them will require some kind of treatment. And as many as one in three men will probably need surgery.

It may come as a surprise to you that, in spite of these alarming statistics, there are very few men who know anything at all about their prostate gland. Most men don't know where it is, what it is, what it does, or what can happen when it goes wrong.

According to a recent MORI poll, only 32 per cent of men in the UK know anything about their prostate gland at all. Yet ignoring the existence of the prostate gland can actually be a foolish – even a dangerous – thing to do.

The animal kingdom

Most male animals have some kind of prostate gland, but animal prostate glands differ greatly from human prostate glands. Most mammalian non-human prostates are very different from human ones. Some animals actually have not one gland, but two or three of them. The fact that animal prostates are so different from human ones means that it is particularly difficult for scientists to conduct research into the prostate. It is only possible to induce either benign enlargement or prostate cancer in very few animals – rats, mice, dogs and guinea-pigs being the only ones.

IN IGNORANCE

Most men will probably have heard it mentioned in the news. They will have heard about famous sufferers of prostate problems – Harold Macmillan, President Ronald Reagan, Australian Prime Minister Bob Hawke, President François Mitterand, Chancellor Helmut Kohl, Frank Zappa and Roger Moore are just seven names that spring to mind. They may also have heard friends or relatives discussing the problems experienced by some elderly relative of theirs.

But by the time they reach their 50s, their 60s, and still more their 70s, the prostate will probably have taken on a more sinister meaning. They will realise by now that, if they haven't already experienced any problems their chances of finishing life without doing so are pretty slim indeed.

Given this unpalatable fact, it makes sense for men to get to know a bit about their prostate gland and what can happen to it. A man who has some understanding of his body, his symptoms and what they mean will be equipped to ask his doctor the right questions if and when the time comes. The informed patient is more likely to gain the respect of his doctor than the total ignoramus, and to enable doctor and patient to form a constructive equal-sided relationship. That, in turn, will give the patient the confidence he needs, especially if he is facing the uncertainties of an illness.

No man can afford to ignore his prostate gland.

The origins of the word

The Greek words from which the word 'prostate' was derived by 16th-century French surgeon Ambroise Paré suggest that it played the role of 'doorkeeper' to the bladder.

WHERE IT IS LOCATED

The prostate is located just below the bladder and in front of the rectum.

It encircles the outlet of the bladder, which is called the urethra, in rather the same way as the cuff encircles the arm during the measurement of blood pressure.

WHAT IT LOOKS LIKE

The prostate gland is small and solid, about the size and shape of a large chestnut. It weighs only a few grams at birth, when it is about the size of a garden pea, and then gains weight as it becomes larger through adolescence. Its weight in an adult man is about 20g. It measures between 1 and 1½ inches in width.

HOW THE PROSTATE CHANGES WITH AGE

The prostate gland begins to enlarge to its adult size at puberty, as a result of the effect of the male hormones, or androgens. It stops enlarging around the age of 20. The prostate rarely causes problems before the age of 30.

In most men, the prostate gland starts to enlarge naturally again after the age of about 50, which is when it often begins to cause the majority of problems. It obviously needs to be located in very close proximity to the urethra because the prostate secretions are discharged into the urethra, but the fact that it actually encircles the urethra in quite this way seems to be a serious design fault in the male anatomy. It is because of this that, as it enlarges with advancing age, it has a tendency to squeeze the urethra and to interfere with the flow of urine.

THE FUNCTIONS OF THE PROSTATE GLAND

The prostate's role in the male body is a curious one. It is not essential for life. It is not even essential for reproduction, though it plays some part in the reproductive process.

The prostate gland is not actually one single gland, but is made up of millions of tiny tubular glands, which are arranged in five lobes: two lateral, a middle, a posterior, and an anterior. The inner zone produces secretions that help keep the lining of the urethra moist; and the outer zone secretes a thin milky fluid, which is discharged into the urethra on ejaculation and makes up between 30 and 40 per cent of semen. Prostatic fluid is therefore an important component of the seminal fluid and provides vital nutrients for sperm.

The prostate gland also contains muscle and fibre cells. These help the gland to contract and to squeeze the secretions of the prostate into the urethra.

Exactly why the prostate gland exists is not really understood.

For further details about the little that we do know of its function, see below.

THE URETHRA

The prostate gland fits like a collar around the urethra, which is the tube that carries urine through the penis to outside the body.

The urethra also carries the semen and sperm during the act of ejaculation.

Sperm are produced in the testes. They are stored in the epididymis, or they can also be temporarily stored at the top of the vasa deferentia, which are the tubes leading from the testes to the ejaculatory ducts which empty into the urethra inside the prostate gland. When a man becomes sexually excited, sperm are pumped up through the vasa deferentia. Then, when a man reaches orgasm, contractions of the seminal vesicles and prostate muscles forces all the available fluid – that is sperm, the fluid from the seminal vesicles situated at the base of the bladder, and the secretions from the prostate gland – to pour into the urethra. Ejaculation then occurs, which is when the muscles surrounding the urethra contract to expel the semen from the penis.

A SUMMARY OF ITS FUNCTIONS

Ignorant as we are about what the prostate gland actually does in the male body, it is known to do the following things:

- It secretes fluids that make up between 30 and 40 per cent of semen. They are added to the seminal fluid while it is collecting at the start of the urethra, a few seconds before ejaculation.
- It secretes certain nutrients that are thought to nourish sperm and keep it healthy. These include zinc, amino acids, citric acid, vitamins and sugars. These nutrients are not necessary for fertilisation, sperm that have not come into contact with prostate fluid can still fertilise an egg. So although it undoubtedly has some influence on male fertility (it helps sperm swim towards the egg and makes the cervix open a little so that sperm can swim through it), it is by no means absolutely indispensable.
- Prostatic fluid contains some substances that neutralise bacteria.
- It helps direct semen outwards during ejaculation. This prevents sperm from refluxing up into the bladder.

- It contains the substances that give semen its characteristic smell.

- It secretes certain enzymes, such as acid phosphatase and prostatic specific antigen (PSA), which give semen its fluidity. It is this that helps sperm to swim.

- It secretes prostaglandins, which are hormone-like chemicals. These have a certain effect on the female genital tract. They make the neck of the womb, or cervix, open a little so that sperm can swim through it into the uterus more easily, and are therefore thought to be important in the process of fertilisation. The fact that the prostatic fluid is believed to be ejaculated in the first contraction of orgasm, just before the bulk of the semen from the seminal vesicles, would appear to support this theory. Prostaglandins are also thought to make the female genital tract contract, which may encourage sperm to be drawn in towards the egg.

- It is the site at which the male sex hormone testosterone – made by the testicles – is broken down.

DISPELLING MYTHS

Given the fact that no one knows a great deal about the role of the prostate, and given the fact that men, in general, seem to have a natural lack of curiosity about their own bodies, it is hardly surprising that so many people have a very distorted idea of what the prostate gland actually does.

Some people have a vague notion that it has something to do with reproduction, and assume that when it goes wrong it therefore causes a reproductive problem. This is not so, however, and the problem is rather to do with the effect of the enlarged or ageing gland on the exit from the bladder.

Some men assume, too, that the prostate is responsible in some way for the production of urine. This belief stems from the fact that, when it becomes enlarged, it makes them urinate more often. But there is no connection at all between the prostate and the kidneys. It is not the manufacture of urine that is the problem, but the exit of urine from the bladder. This is because when the prostate enlarges – for whatever reason – it exerts pressure on the urethra and on the neck of the bladder, thereby restricting the flow of urine.

It is useful to understand what the prostate gland does and what it means when it goes wrong. A lot of men who have problems with the flow of urine and find it difficult to cope with an increased frequency of urination think they can rectify the problem by cutting down on their fluid intake. But this is not only useless, it can also be dangerous. People who have an obstructed bladder should actually drink more, not less, even though this may mean 'going' more often. This is because, if there is any residual urine left in the bladder, this may become infected unless it is regularly diluted with a fresh supply of urine.

Nor should you try to hold out for as long as possible before emptying your bladder. You will empty your bladder more efficiently when you are not in a hurry.

2 Disorders of the Prostate

There can be very few disorders associated with any one particular organ that occur as commonly as prostate problems. If you think about it, all men are at risk, which accounts for about 50 per cent of the population. In turn, it is estimated by experts in the field that around half of all men over the age of 50 have symptoms that can be blamed on the prostate.

In total, that accounts for a very large proportion of the overall population.

THE MAIN DISORDERS

The main disorders that can affect the prostate are infections and tumours – the majority of which are benign rather than malignant.

There are three main things that can go wrong with the pros tate gland. These are:

- Prostatitis.
- Benign prostatic hyperplasia (BPH).
- Prostate cancer.

PROSTATITIS

Prostatitis is an umbrella term covering several disorders. In this condition, the prostate gland becomes inflamed due to infection. It is extremely common, particularly between the ages of 30 and 50, and it is estimated that as many as one in three men suffers from prostatitis at some time. It can be present for many years without producing any symptoms, and then suddenly flare up for no apparent reason. It may be acute or chronic.

Post-mortem studies have shown that one in five men under the age of 40 has had chronic prostatitis at some time, while as many as three out of five men over the age of 40 have had this condition. This suggests that chronic inflammation of the prostate gland may occur without producing any symptoms. Chronic non-bacterial prostatitis is most common between the ages of 30 and 50.

Acute or chronic?

An acute disorder comes on suddenly. It may or may not be severe, but is usually of short duration. A chronic condition, on the other hand, is one that persists for a long time (sometimes in spite of treatment).

What causes it?

Prostatitis is often caused by a bacterial infection that has spread from the intestines. These find their way into the urinary system, either through the urethra or through the bloodstream or lymphatic fluids.

Sometimes there is a link with the organisms that cause a sexually-transmitted disease, such as gonorrhoea or chlamydia. Sometimes, too, the fungus that causes thrush (Candida) is responsible.

What you can do about it

Prostatitis – both chronic and acute – is usually treated by a prolonged course of the appropriate antibiotic. Treatment can be difficult, particularly of chronic prostatitis, and infection may persist in the prostate, in spite of treatment. When this happens, the condition may tend to recur.

AN ENLARGED PROSTATE

An enlarged prostate is also known as benign prostatic hyperplasia (BPH), or as benign prostatic hypertrophy.

The prostate gland enlarges naturally as a man gets older, particularly after the age of 50. This happens because of an increase in the number of cells present in the prostate gland. As the number of cells increases, so the prostate gland gets correspondingly bigger. This process is known as hyperplasia.

The part of the prostate that causes the problem is the central part, close to the urethra.

It most commonly causes symptoms after the age of 50 or so, and according to a recent survey conducted by Professor William Garraway in Scotland (*Lancet*, 1991), one in three men over the age of 50 is reckoned to experience symptoms. It becomes increasingly common with advancing age. By the age of 60, for example, around 60 per cent of men have clinical symptoms; by the age of 70, around 70 per cent have symptoms; and so on.

A lot of men never consult their doctor about the symptoms of an enlarged prostate because they are too embarrassed to do so. Instead, they suffer in silence and put up with an ever-worsening condition.

The symptoms develop slowly over the years. The result of this is that many men assume that they are just an inevitable part of the ageing process, and do not seek medical advice or treatment until much later.

Some men are lucky enough never to get any symptoms. In the great majority of men, however, because the prostate gland is wrapped round the urethra – the tube through which urine passes when a man urinates – an enlarged prostate causes the urethra to become compressed. The resulting symptoms, which are a combination of urinary outflow obstruction, are known as prostatism.

What causes it?

The cause of prostate enlargement is not altogether clear. What is

17

clear, however, is that an enlarged prostate is a male hormone dependent disorder in that its growth is stimulated by androgens and, in particular, by testosterone. What is not clear, though, is why it should suddenly enlarge at the age of 50 or more, when testosterone levels tend to fall.

The fact that the cause of an enlarged prostate is not certain and is, in any case, beyond our control, means that, unfortunately, there is no clear advice that can be given on how best to avoid prostate enlargement. The good thing about this, though, is that there is no need to reproach yourself if you suffer from prostate enlargement – no cause for such thoughts as 'If only I'd . . . ', or 'If only I hadn't . . . ', or whatever.

What you can do about it

Drug treatment – such as alpha-blockers and 5-alpha-reductase inhibitors – is recommended for many sufferers, particularly if their condition is not too severe. Many doctors, however, feel that surgery is the only solution to an enlarged prostate, especially in severe cases. As a result and as the Department of Health knows only too well, the annual cost of hospital care and surgery for an enlarged prostate is extremely high.

There are, however, other solutions. An enlarged prostate will often respond well to alternative treatments (see Chapter 9). It is important to realise this because waiting lists for surgery can be very long, and in any case surgery can result in complications.

PROSTATE CANCER

According to the Cancer Research Campaign, prostate cancer accounts for some 8,000 deaths in the UK each year, and for at least 149,000 deaths each year throughout the world. It is the second most common fatal cancer in men after lung cancer. It kills some four times as many men as cervical cancer kills women, and yet this statistic – unlike those concerning cervical cancer – is hardly ever mentioned, and certainly never hits the headlines in quite the same way. Many people, including a lot of men, often know much more about cervical cancer in women than prostate cancer in men.

The symptoms of benign prostate enlargement are similar to those of prostate cancer, which is just one very good reason for not sweeping them under the carpet and for taking them to the doctor. It is possible for an enlarged prostate to be malignant, but it is much more likely to be benign. You should always keep things in perspective and never fear the worst.

Prostate cancer usually occurs over the age of 55, though it can in some cases occur much earlier. According to the Cancer Research Campaign, some 14,000 new cases are diagnosed each year, and one in every eleven men will probably develop signs of prostate cancer at some point in their lives. That makes it almost as common as breast cancer in women, yet it doesn't get quite the same press coverage, and it doesn't cause quite the same alarm. Men are significantly less aware of the potential problem they carry around in their bodies than women are of the possibility of breast cancer, the fear of which is all too real for many women throughout their lives.

But if men knew more about the signs of prostate cancer revealed during post-mortem examinations, they might not be so complacent. These reveal an alarmingly high incidence of prostate cancer. Among men aged between 50 and 60 years, 10-30 per cent show evidence of cancer when the prostate is examined under the microscope. In men aged between 70 and 80, the figure is still more astonishing: as many as 50-70 per cent show the same signs.

In most cases, prostate cancer is what is known as a 'silent' disease. That is to say that it never causes significant problems and is often never even diagnosed. The chances are that a man who has prostate cancer will probably never even know he has it, and is unlikely to die of it – he will die of something else first.

The Royal College of Surgeons completed a study of 5,500 prostate cases in 1995. One of the most striking messages to emerge from this is that if you have prostate cancer and *live long enough*, it will kill you, but you are unlikely to live long enough for this to happen.

A report from the Office of Health Economics, also in 1995, would seem to support this view. It quotes a study showing that 70 per cent of men over the age of 80 have prostate cancer, but that only 0.5 per cent die from it.

What causes it?

Like a great many cancers, cancer of the prostate is known to run in families. If a close relative has had cancer of the prostate, a man's risk of developing the disease seems to be a lot higher than that of a man who does not have any family history of the disease.

Another factor that seems to be involved is diet. The typical UK diet, which is usually low in green vegetables, fruit and pulses and high in fats – may well be a contributing factor.

What you can do about it

Prostate cancer may be treated in a number of ways, depending on how early the cancer has been discovered and on how far it has spread. If it has spread beyond the prostate gland, treatment will probably be aimed at controlling the condition rather than attempting to cure it.

Treatment may be done in several ways. These are:

- The surgical removal of the prostate, which is known as pros-tatectomy (see Chapter 7).
- Radiotherapy.

If the cancer has spread to other parts of the body, patients may benefit from reducing their level of the male hormone testosterone. This can be done by:

- Surgical removal of the testes (orchidectomy).
- The administration of hormonal drugs.
- Radiotherapy, which shrinks the prostate gland or relieves the pain of secondary bone cancer, if it exists.

CONSULTING YOUR DOCTOR

The main thing to bear in mind is that when you suspect that there is something wrong – and no matter what that is – you should always consult your doctor.

Although at least one in three men over the age of 50 experiences at least one – and maybe more – of the uncomfortable symptoms of an enlarged prostate (*Lancet*, 1991), some of which can be very unpleasant as well as having a dramatic effect on their lives, only six out of ten of them will actually go to their doctor. They may be embarrassed to talk about anything concerning their urinary habits; they may be frightened of being accused of wasting their doctor's time; or they may think that their symptoms are nothing more than an inevitable part of the normal ageing process and therefore don't warrant a visit to the doctor.

They may also be frightened of being ill. A lot of men, while making a tremendous fuss every time they have a cold, are actually reluctant to visit the doctor, particularly if they fear that they have something badly, or dangerously, wrong with their health.

You should never be too frightened to see the doctor. He won't invent a serious problem where there isn't one, and if there is one he may well be able to do something about it.

What your doctor will do

The doctor will want to know all your symptoms, and it is always worth making a list of these before you go to the surgery so as not to forget to mention anything. If you're embarrassed by talking about your symptoms, you might even hand your list to your doctor and ask him to read it. Make a note of any questions you want to ask – there's nothing worse than visiting the doctor and then remembering later that you've forgotten to ask the one thing that you really wanted to know.

The doctor will take a general medical history, with particular reference to any serious familial diseases such as diabetes, heart

THE COMPLETE PROSTATE HANDBOOK

disease or haemophilia, and any drugs you are taking. He will also want to know any important changes in your health that you have noticed recently, such as general fatigue or lower back pain, which may not seem to you to be at all relevant but which may be important to the doctor in his search for a diagnosis.

And then, of course, the doctor will also want to know all about your current symptoms. He will want to know, in particular, anything relating to your urinary habits. How high/strong is your flow of urine? Do you have any difficulties urinating – either starting or stopping? Do you experience any pain on urinating? How often do you urinate? Do you have to get up at night to empty your bladder? Are your symptoms having a major effect on your life, and if so in what way? And since when have you been experiencing these symptoms?

You may feel more comfortable seeing a male doctor than a woman. If that is so, this should not cause any problem. Most practices have doctors of both sexes and you can generally choose whether to see a man or a woman. Your doctor will not be unsympathetic to your expressing a preference of this sort.

Don't be embarrassed to talk to your doctor about your urinary habits. Remember, he's heard it all before. He's not embarrassed and there is no need for you to be either.

Injury

In spite of the fact that the prostate gland is so well hidden, tucked away as it is inside a man's body, it can nevertheless be injured by a blow between the buttocks. It can also be irritated by any sort of over-firm, continuous pressure. A long-distance lorry driver, for example, can suffer from this as a result of having a badly sprung seat.

Enlarged prostate and cancer of the prostate

The early symptoms of an enlarged prostate and cancer of the prostate are so similar as to be practically indistinguishable. But they are quite different disorders, and an enlarged prostate, otherwise known as benign prostatic hyperplasia, does not become cancerous.

Some people think that benign enlargement must be some kind of pre-cancerous condition, and that this is why surgeons are in such a hurry to remove it. But this is not true. Benign enlargement tends to occur in the inner part of the prostate – the bit that actually encircles the urethra – and works its way gradually outwards. Cancer of the prostate, on the other hand, starts in the outer part of the gland, which explains why it can be felt during a rectal examination. There is absolutely no evidence that benign enlargement can turn cancerous.

3 The Prostate in Sexual Activity

The prostate is part of the male reproductive system and supplies part of the seminal fluid. It is not essential for the man's sexuality, though, nor even for his ability to reproduce.

When a man's prostate is removed, male sexuality is not normally affected. His sex drive is intact, and his ability to achieve and maintain an erection is unchanged.

SEMINAL FLUID

Sperm makes up only a small part of the seminal fluid. In fact most of the fluid you ejaculate isn't sperm at all. Most of the fluid consists mainly of secretions from a number of glands. The largest of these glands is the prostate.

The various secretions from these glands probably serve the purpose of providing the sperm with a greater motility after they have been ejaculated, which stimulates their activity and enables them to move towards the egg.

It is thought by some people that the prostate also has a lot to do with the feeling that an orgasm gives you. When a man has an orgasm, sperm fluid from the seminal vesicles and the secretions from the prostate all mix together as semen at the top of the urethra, just below the bladder. A man gets an intensely pleasurable sensation when the semen floods down the urethra into the penis. He also gets a pleasurable feeling when the semen squirts out of the penis and into the tight region of a woman's vagina. The prostate gland can be felt, as a man's orgasm proceeds, to contract rhythmically, which some people believe to be very much an integral part of the pleasure he experiences on orgasm.

What prostate fluid contains

- Water.
- Salts.
- Minerals.
- Proteins.
- Antibodies.
- Enzymes.
- Citric acid.
- Fats.
- Prostaglandins, which are hormone-like chemicals.

PROSTATIC DISEASE

Prostatic disease can have an effect not only on the urinary system, but also on the reproductive system. The male reproductive and urinary systems are, of course, closely linked, if only because they share the same exit route – the penis – or, to be more exact, the urethra which runs through the centre of the penis.

The prostate gland is the site at which the male sex hormone testosterone, which is made by the testicles, is broken down. It is here that it then forms another hormone called dihydrotestosterone (DHT). The conversion is controlled by an enzyme called 5-alpha-reductase.

In a study conducted by Imperato-McGinley (*Science*, 1974), the males in an obscure tribe in the Dominican Republic are deficient in 5-alpha-reductase and are often mistaken for girls until they reach puberty. Until then, they have a very small penis and scrotum, which suddenly enlarge at puberty, along with the development of a deep voice. These males only ever develop a very small prostate gland, they never go bald, and they do not suffer from acne.

It is this genetic deficiency in 5-alpha-reductase that has enabled researchers to comprehend the role played by dihydrotestosterone in the enlargement of the prostate gland.

Testosterone

As well as prostate enlargement, the male hormone testosterone also has several other effects on the male body.

These include the following:

- The growth of the penis.
- The growth of testes.
- The production of sperm .
- A deeper voice.
- The growth of facial and body hair.
- The male sex drive.
- Bone growth.
- Strength.
- Acne.
- Baldness

A MAN'S GREATEST FEARS

One of man's greatest fears on seeing a urologist and considering the prospect of a prostatectomy is what effect this will have on his sexuality. The idea of having any sexual organ tampered with by a surgeon is very frightening for most men, who worry that it may have a deleterious effect on their sex lives.

Many men are so frightened that their prostate problems will affect their sex lives, particularly if they have to have an operation, that they put off going to the doctor. And even when they do eventually go to the doctor, they may be too embarrassed to discuss sexual matters. Sex is something that all too many men find difficult – if not impossible – to talk about with their doctor.

But this is foolish. It is only by talking the matter over with their doctor that they will find their fears were groundless and that they can therefore be reassured.

The doctor's role

To make matters worse, some doctors and urologists are sometimes insensitive on this subject. It is quite wrong of them to assume that their patients are too old to be interested in sex. Sex can play an important role in the lives of many men until well into old age, and they should treat their fears as real and serious.

A man who is due to have a prostatectomy should not just fret about this in secret, he should talk to his doctors about it – his GP, his consultant, his surgeon. Most importantly, the doctor should respect his fears, and him for coming to air them with him.

It's not easy for any man to do this, and if he succeeds in overcoming his reluctance to do so, the doctor should recognise what that has cost him. If the doctor reacts badly, it might have catastrophic effects: it might just send him scuttling back to his burrow, his pride injured, and he might never be able to take the risk again.

Only when both doctor and patient can talk about this calmly, sensibly, realistically, will the patient be reassured that it will have no effect on his sexuality – neither on his libido, nor his ability to obtain or maintain an erection, nor on his performance.

Retrograde ejaculation

What it may well do, however, is cause him to be infertile after the operation (see Chapters 7 and 8).

Even a man who has no intention of becoming a father again may find the idea of losing his potential to be a father very distressing. A man may find this emasculating, as if it were questioning his manhood. He's only lost his ability to procreate, not his sexuality, but this can have a devastating effect on him. This is reminiscent of a woman who regrets the loss of her womb after a hysterectomy, even though she is beyond childbearing, and feels she has lost her femininity.

A doctor should have the sensitivity to talk to his patient about this. Only with patience and understanding can he help him come to terms with his feelings of fear and loss.

Retrograde ejaculation will not make a man impotent, nor – in most cases – will it prevent him from having orgasms. It will, however, make the sensation of orgasm a different one – and, in all honesty, probably not as good a one. Some women, too, are disappointed by the new feeling of a 'dry' climax in their male partner.

These changes in a man's sexuality should be addressed beforehand. He should be told what to expect. A sensitive doctor will also help a couple come to terms with their new-found sexuality.

Impotence

It is possible, though by no means certain – nor even common – that prostatectomy may cause impotence. Some men are frightened that it might have this effect, probably because they have heard tales of the old perineal prostate operation (which is hardly ever done nowadays) or the radical prostatectomy in which the entire prostate, including the capsule in which it is enclosed, is removed (sometimes performed for prostate cancer). In both these operations, the nerves supplying the penis were sometimes cut, which led to a man's impotentence. If these operations are done today, it is usually – though not always – possible to avoid cutting these nerves. The problem of impotence is therefore unlikely but it may arise.

If a man is very frightened that the operation may lead to impotence, he may actually experience a kind of psychological impotence afterwards. This underlines how important it is for a man to be reassured before the operation. If a psychological problem does occur, a counsellor or sex therapist should be able to deal with it.

An excuse to avoid sex

In spite of all the evidence that prostate surgery has no effect at all on a man's sexuality (other than retrograde ejaculation), it does occasionally seem to happen. An obvious explanation for this is that some men may use surgery as an excuse to avoid sex, which they had stopped enjoying ages ago anyway. Occasionally, if a man is not in very good health, a prostate operation – which is, after all, a major operation requiring a long convalescence period – may be enough to push his sexuality over the edge.

Generally, though, most men do not have any problems with their sex lives after the operation. In fact, a man may actually find that his sex life has greatly improved since he had his prostatectomy, if only because he now has full control of his bladder.

AN EROGENOUS ZONE

Some people believe that the prostate gland is a highly erogenous zone and that awareness of this can greatly heighten a man's sexual pleasure.

Many sex therapists consider that the man's prostate gland is the equivalent to a woman's G-spot. In fact the female G-spot and the male prostate gland are located in very much the same position.

In order to find a man's prostate gland, proceed in the following way:

* With the man lying face down on the bed, with a couple of pillows under his hips, insert a well-lubricated finger into his rectum, palm facing downwards.
* You should feel his prostate as a firm mass, about the size of a large chestnut. Stroke it with your fingers.
* Be guided by what he tells you. This should feel very pleasurable and produce intense sexual sensations. Ask him how it feels, and do what he likes best.
* Keep on stroking his prostate until he ejaculates. Many men

ejaculate while this is being done without ever having an erection.

- An alternative position to this is with the man on his back and his legs drawn right up. In this position, the prostate can be felt on the front wall of the rectum.

A woman's objections

Some women object to doing this to their lover because they are frightened that it will be messy. It may be, but the lower part of the rectum is usually empty anyway, so there should not be a problem.

One way of dealing with this is for the woman to use a latex finger stall, which is available from the chemist to cover a finger that has an open wound on it. This is intended to keep the finger waterproof.

Whatever you use – a naked finger or a finger with a finger stall – you should wash it carefully afterwards. The anus is a breeding ground for bacteria, and it pays to be careful about hygiene.

Some women are frightened that they might hurt their lover when they do this. It is true that the anal area is very sensitive and they should therefore always be careful. They should, in particular, make sure that they do not have a sharp or jagged nail on the finger they use to do this.

They should be careful, too, not do this if they have any open cuts on the finger used, in case of the transmission of HIV or hepatitis B.

4 Prostatitis

Prostatitis is a catch-all expression covering various types of inflammation of the prostate. It is not as serious as enlargement of the prostate, and especially not as serious as cancer of the prostate. It can, however, be a very difficult condition to treat and can sometimes drag on for several years.

In prostatitis, the tiny glands in the prostate become infected, inflamed or clogged – either with thickened secretions or with small gravel-like stones. As we have seen in Chapter 1, the prostate is a complex system of glands, cells, tubules and ducts. Once infection gets a hold in this complicated network, it is hardly surprising that it can be very difficult to eradicate.

Even when it has been treated – and even when it seems as though it has been successfully treated – it can still come back. And in the absence of successful treatment, it can flare up for years, with depressing regularity.

THREE TYPES

There are three main types of prostatitis. These are:
- Acute bacterial infection.
- Chronic infection, which may be bacterial or non-bacterial.
- Prostatodynia, which may cause the symptoms of prostate pain without any obvious signs of inflammation or infection.

DIAGNOSIS OF PROSTATITIS

Prostatitis is sometimes difficult to diagnose. In general, the person best qualified to diagnose prostatitis is a doctor specialising in urology or genito-urinary medicine.

Your doctor may refer you to a special genito-urinary (GU) clinic. This does not mean that your doctor suspects that you are suffering from a sexually-transmitted disease. It simply means that genito-urinary clinics have the best experience and equipment to investigate and treat your symptoms. The staff are used to dealing with this kind of problem, and will do so sympathetically and in confidence, so you have no need to feel embarrassed.

You are likely to have a number of tests as part of the investigation of your symptoms. These may include some, or all, of the following:

- A digital rectal examination, which means that the doctor inserts a lubricated gloved finger into the rectum and gently palpates, or feels, the prostate through the front wall of the rectum, which lies against the back of the gland. If you have prostatitis, the prostate will feel boggy, soft and tender. A digital rectal examination should not hurt, though it may be uncomfortable if the prostate is inflamed and therefore tender to the touch. A lot of men are embarrassed to have one, but they shouldn't be: doctors are used to doing this and have a very matter-of-fact attitude to it.

- Swabs from the end of the penis, which are taken by gently inserting a sterile cotton bud into the end of the penis and taking any fresh discharge.

- Urine tests to check for cloudiness, signs of protein or blood, and threads of cellular material, which are then examined under the microscope for pus cells or bacteria.

- Urine cultures to see if any bacteria grow, which should also distinguish between infection in different parts of the urinary tract.

- A blood test to check for a raised white cell count.

- Routine screening for sexually-transmitted diseases such as chlamydia.

- The doctor will look for a discharge from the penis, and for signs of inflammation and soreness both on the penis and in the testicles.

THE RISKS

If prostatitis is untreated, or if drug treatment is unsuccessful, there is a risk that the prostate gland may become full of pus. Not surprisingly, this can have dreadful consequences.

It may eventually burst, releasing pus into the urethra, which will discharge from the tip of the penis. And it may also result in severe infection elsewhere in the urinary tract.

ACUTE BACTERIAL INFECTION

This is an uncommon complaint. It is usually caused by bacteria from the intestines. These find their way into the urinary system, either through the urethra or through the bloodstream or lymphatic fluids.

Sometimes there is a link with organisms that cause a sexually-transmitted disease, such as gonorrhoea or chlamydia. Sometimes, too, the fungus that causes thrush (Candida) is responsible.

Symptoms

These can happen suddenly and can include one or several of the following:

- Feeling generally under the weather.
- Chills or fever.
- An aching feeling around the thighs and genitals.
- A deep pain in the perineum, which is the area between the pouch containing the testicles, known as the scrotum, and the anus.
- Low back pain.
- Pain in the lower abdomen.
- Pain on passing water.
- Blood in the urine, which is known as haematuria.
- Difficulty in passing water.

- Increased frequency of passing water.
- Urine may be cloudy or smelly.
- Pain on ejaculation.

Diagnosis

The doctor will probably perform a digital rectal examination by inserting a lubricated gloved finger into the rectum. He will then feel the prostate through the wall of the rectum. If a man has prostatitis, the prostate will probably feel hot, swollen and tender.

The doctor will then do a series of tests on a sample of urine and on urethral secretions obtained after massaging the prostate gland, in order to investigate the cause of the infection.

Treatment

Acute bacterial prostatitis, when symptoms come on suddenly, is the most dramatic form of the disease, but it is also the form that responds best to treatment. A prolonged course of antibiotic tablets is prescribed. This is usually for at least four weeks. Acute infection responds well to antibiotics, probably because the intense inflammation allows the drugs to penetrate into the interior of the gland. Symptoms should begin to show some improvement within the first few days.

Sometimes, though, infection may persist in the prostate, in spite of treatment, and it is necessary to have careful follow-up treatment to make sure that the condition has cleared up. If this does not happen, the condition may tend to recur and chronic prostatitis will usually result.

Occasionally, though rarely, infection may cause the gland to swell sufficiently for the urethra to be squeezed shut. This causes urinary outflow obstruction. It necessitates urgent admission to hospital, where urinary flow is eased by inserting a catheter directly into the bladder through the abdomen under local anaesthetic. With rest and the administration of antibiotics, the infection will usually clear up well in only a few days.

CHRONIC PROSTATITIS

Chronic prostatitis is more common than acute prostatitis, but is much more difficult to eradicate.

There are two types of chronic prostatitis, which can be bacterial or non-bacterial.

Chronic bacterial prostatitis

Micro-organisms can enter the prostate gland, where they set up a localised infection with pus and perhaps with abscesses. Swelling occurs rapidly and this traps the bacteria in the gland, as the usual drainage channels become blocked off.

Prostatic secretions may coat the offending bacteria, which then harden to form tiny stones, or crystals. This protects them from being attacked by the body's immune system or by antibiotics. This explains the repeated flare-ups that tend to occur in chronic bacterial prostatitis.

This means, too, that the condition can be difficult to treat successfully. Some sufferers may even be unlucky enough to suffer from recurrent symptoms throughout their lives.

Symptoms

These vary from one person to another. They may include any, or several, of the following:

- Frequency in passing water.
- Pain on passing water.
- Pain in the prostate, genitals or rectum.
- Swelling of the testes.
- Lower back pain.
- Watery discharge from the penis.
- Pain on ejaculation.
- Blood in the semen.

- Premature ejaculation.
- If the doctor feels the prostate during a digital rectal examination, it may feel boggy, soft and squelchy.

Fertility

There is some evidence that chronic bacterial prostatitis may impair male fertility. This may probably be true in all cases of prostatitis, but seems to be especially true of chronic bacterial prostatitis. Analysis of the prostatic fluid of men with chronic bacterial prostatitis has shown significant changes in both the physical properties and the chemical constituents of the fluid. It is thought that these changes may well affect the quality of the semen, and thus the level of fertility. It is not unusual for doctors to hear the wives of men with chronic bacterial prostatitis complain that they are finding it difficult to become pregnant. A sperm count and sperm quality assessment can be done to find out how much a man's fertility has been affected.

Chronic non-bacterial prostatitis

This is a complaint in which inflammation is present without any signs of infection. In other words, prostate secretions contain white pus cells, but no bacteria.

It is not known exactly what causes chronic non-bacterial prostatitis, but several theories have been suggested. One is that it is caused by abnormal emptying of the bladder, which forces urine into the prostate channels and ducts, where it causes irritation and inflammation. This may be triggered, or aggravated, if a man jogs or plays any strenuous sport on a full bladder.

Another theory is that some men produce thicker prostate secretions, which are perhaps more acid then normal. These secretions are unable to drain away through the narrow ducts and therefore build up to cause irritation and swelling.

Symptoms

The most common symptoms of chronic non-bacterial prostatitis are:

- Frequency in passing water.
- Pain on passing water.
- Pain or ache in the prostate, genitals or rectum.
- Lower back pain, especially after sexual intercourse.
- Discharge from the urethra, especially after intercourse.

Treatment

Any chronic infection is difficult to treat, particularly when inflammation and swellings trap the infection inside the gland.

In the case of chronic bacterial prostatitis, a course of the appropriate antibiotic, depending on which bacterium is responsible for the condition, will be prescribed for at least six weeks. Sometimes antibiotics may be required for as long as three months, or even longer.

Chronic non-bacterial prostatitis can be treated with a natural food supplement derived from rye pollen extracts, which has been shown to reduce inflammation, irritation and swelling, though improvement may not be apparent for at least three months and full recovery may take as long as six months or even more. Swelling, inflammation and pain may be helped by anti-inflammatory pain-killers such as ibuprofen.

Self-help

Chronic non-bacterial prostatitis is sometimes relieved by an increased frequency of ejaculation. This can be brought about through intercourse, of course, but if this does not happen it may equally be brought about by masturbation.

Ejaculation drains the prostate of any excess secretions and causes a temporary increase in blood supply. Both these things help to flush away any toxins.

In some cases, however, an increased frequency of ejaculation only makes the problem worse.

PROSTATODYNIA

This is characterised by the usual symptoms of prostate problems, including pain, but with no evidence of inflammation or infection in the gland. Prostate secretions look perfectly normal and contain no pus cells.

Prostatodynia is surprisingly common and accounts for around one third of all cases where men experience the symptoms of chronic prostatitis.

Symptoms

The symptoms of prostatodynia are therefore similar to those of chronic prostatitis. They may often also include psychosexual problems.

Symptoms include the following:

- Frequency in passing water, sometimes with associated pain.
- Pain in the prostate, genitals or rectum.
- Swelling of the testes.
- Lower back pain.
- Watery discharge from the penis.
- Blood in the semen (haemospermia).
- Premature ejaculation.
- Pain on erection.
- Pain on ejaculation.
- Low sex drive.
- A diminished volume of semen.
- Impotence.
- If the doctor feels the prostate during a digital rectal examination, it may feel boggy, soft and squelchy.

Treatment

Prostatodynia can be difficult to treat. Painkillers are not usually helpful.

Some doctors have labelled prostatodynia as a psychosexual problem and advise counselling. It is, however, likely to have a physical cause, such as spasm of the pelvic muscles, which may be brought on by stress and anxiety. In this case, tranquillisers may be prescribed in order to reduce muscular spasm in the gland, though it is not a good idea to take these in the long-term as they can become addictive.

Recent studies have suggested that prostate pain can be relieved by microwave hyperthermia. The technique was originally developed at the Beilinson Medical Centre, Petah Tiqva, in Israel in the early 1980s and is now attracting a lot of interest in other countries. This entails warming the prostate gland from body temperature (37°C/98.6°F) to 42.5°C/180.5°F by a special instrument which is inserted into the back passage. This increases the blood supply and accelerates the body's natural healing reactions. An hour's treatment is usually given weekly for six weeks.

Other treatments that have been tried for prostatodynia include:

- Acupuncture.
- Laser irradiation.
- Muscle-relaxant drugs, such as diazepam.
- Antispasmodic drugs.

Self-help

As in chronic non-bacterial prostatitis, symptoms may be worsened when ejaculation is infrequent, in which case the pain may be caused by prostatic gland engorgement. Symptoms may therefore be relieved by an increased frequency of ejaculation, as a result of either intercourse or masturbation. Ejaculation drains the prostate of any excess secretions and causes a temporary increase in blood supply, both of which help to flush out any toxins.

In some cases, however, an increased frequency of ejaculation only makes the problem worse.

Sitting in a hot bath for half an hour can help to warm up the prostate gland. Relaxation techniques may also be used to relax the muscles and as an alternative to muscle-relaxant drugs.

The combination of regular exercise and a high-fibre diet will help keep the bowels regular, which is particularly important for men suffering from prostatodynia. This is of special benefit to those men who sit at a desk for most of the day, as both constant sitting and constipation tend to increase prostate congestion.

Symptoms of prostatodynia may be triggered by the nicotine in cigarettes and by alcohol or caffeine, so it is best to reduce consumption of all three. It may also be advisable to consult an allergy specialist who may be able to identify foods that you should avoid.

Natural treatments

Rye pollen extracts have been shown in clinical trials in Europe to help ease the symptoms of prostatitis, particularly chronic non-bacterial prostatitis and prostatodynia. They reduce inflammation and ease irritation. They may take as long as three months before they show any improvement, which may then continue over the next three months. Rye pollen extracts, such as Cernilton and ProstaBrit, are available from health food stores (see also Naturopathy, Chapter 9).

Prostatitis and sex

If you suffer from prostatitis, it is a good idea to avoid sex, both while you are having symptoms and while you are being treated. This is because, if the problem is one of infection, you may pass this on to a female partner, in which case it may manifest itself as cystitis or vaginal infection.

Your doctor will be able to advise you on when you can resume normal sexual relations.

---

5 Enlarged Prostate

As we have learned, the prostate gland enlarges naturally as a man gets older. It can enlarge from the size of a chestnut to the size of an apple. This happens because of an increase in the number of cells present in the prostate gland, in a process known as hyperplasia.

Some doctors believe that every man over the age of 50 has some degree of prostate enlargement and that it is simply part of the ageing process. This view is supported by routine tests, which show that nearly every man over the age of 50 has some degree of enlargement of the prostate gland.

Prostate enlargement is correctly called benign prostatic hyperplasia (BPH) and is also known as benign prostatic hypertrophy. Benign means that, unlike cancer, it is not malignant, but it does not mean that it is harmless. An enlarged prostate can exist for many years and cause little more than irritation and inconvenience. Left untreated, however, it can cause severe harm.

Enlargement, in itself, does not necessarily cause problems. A lot of growths of prostate tissue are a natural part of the ageing process and are quite harmless. What is not so harmless, though, is when little gristly nodules accumulate, the development of which changes both the size and consistency of the gland. For it is not actually size that matters so much as the consistency of the tissues, which causes the gland to become stiff and inflexible. Sometimes the bladder can compensate for this by becoming stronger and more powerful, but problems occur when the bladder muscles can no longer overcome the resistance caused by the increasingly rigid prostate gland.

This is when the flow of urine becomes badly obstructed – which can have a dramatic and troublesome effect on a man's lifestyle. It is important to realise, however, that you do not have to accept this as an inevitable part of ageing. It isn't – in the sense, at least, that something can almost always be done about it.

NEVER SUFFER IN SILENCE

Because the prostate gland surrounds the urethra, and because it is located so close to the base of the bladder, when it becomes enlarged it can seriously interfere with the normal function of urination. As a result, an enlarged prostate can be both troublesome and inconvenient. It is likely to mean disturbed sleep, interrupted by several visits to the toilet every night; and it will probably mean curtailing social activities because of the need to be near a toilet at all times.

But there is no need to suffer in silence. If you think you have an enlarged prostate, you must see your doctor as soon as possible. It is not an emergency, requiring instant admission to Accident and Emergency, but it does require prompt treatment. As long as it is treated promptly, it can almost always effectively relieve symptoms.

More seriously, an enlarged prostate can have several severe consequences, though these are not common. It can, for example, cause acute urine retention, in which case there is an urgent need for catheterisation – or the insertion of a flexible tube into the bladder under local anaesthetic – which will bring instant relief. In an even more serious case, it can cause trapped urine to flow back up from the bladder, where it will put pressure on the kidneys and may even, in severe cases, lead to kidney failure. This happens only rarely, but its possibility is nevertheless a good reason for taking an enlarged prostate seriously.

WHAT CAUSES AN ENLARGED PROSTATE?

Why the prostate gland gets bigger is not really known. Only two things are certain, and that is that the only people who suffer from an enlarged prostate have two things in common:

- They are male.
- They are getting on in years.

The exact cause of prostate enlargement is not altogether clear. What is clear, is that an enlarged prostate is a male hormone-dependent disorder in that its growth is stimulated by androgens and, in particular, by testosterone. What is not clear, however, is why it should suddenly enlarge at the age of 50 or more, when testosterone levels are falling.

Another possible factor influencing the development of an enlarged prostate includes the sort of diet you eat. A food link is suspected because of the undeniable fact that so many more men suffer from an enlarged prostate in the West than in eastern societies such as China and Japan. It is felt that this may be because western and eastern ways of eating are so different. It is possible that the men in eastern societies are protected by their diet, which relies heavily on soya-based foods such as tofu, and on plant foods such as vegetables and fruit.

Sex hormones

It does seem to be an odd fact that the organs of the body that depend on sex hormones – both male and female – are particularly prone to disorders of growth, which can be either benign or malignant.

This is, for example, that women are prone to both benign and malignant growths in the breasts and the womb – a third of all cancers in women, in fact, affect these organs.

In just this same way, men are prone to enlargement of the prostate gland, which can be either benign or malignant. One tenth of all male cancers, in fact, affect the prostate gland.

Levels of prolactin

The level of the hormone prolactin is known to increase dihydrotestosterone in the prostate gland and thus to encourage prostatic enlargement. Two things that are known to *increase* levels of prolactin, and may therefore contribute to an enlarged prostate, are:

- Stress.
- Beer.

Two things that are known to *reduce* levels of prolactin are:

- Zinc.
- Vitamin B6.

Deficiency of one or both of these nutrients may therefore contribute to prostatic enlargement (see Naturopathy, Chapter 9).

WHO IS AT RISK OF PROSTATE ENLARGEMENT?

The answer to this is anyone and everyone. No one knows of anything that decreases the risk, so there's nothing you can do to minimise your chances. People talk about a prostate-friendly diet (see Chapter 10), and this way of eating is probably good for the general health of everyone – women as well as men, but following this diet in no way guarantees that you will never have anything wrong with your prostate. Sadly, it won't.

SYMPTOMS

Some men never experience any symptoms. Others, however – the great majority, in fact – experience urinary outflow obstruction, known as prostatism, which is caused quite simply by the fact that the prostate gland encircles the urethra. As the prostate gets bigger, so it presses on the urethra, which becomes more or less severely narrowed as a result.

If you think that you have symptoms of an enlarged prostate, see your doctor as soon as you can. Don't wait until symptoms interfere with your lifestyle.

Recognising the symptoms

The symptoms of an enlarged prostate, which are known as prostatism, are purely mechanical. They are rarely troublesome before the age of 55, and affect one in ten elderly males.

Some of these symptoms are due to distortion of the normal anatomy at the base of the bladder, which causes urinary outflow obstruction. Some are caused by irritation to the bladder as it stretches and thickens in an attempt to push urine past the obstruction caused by the prostate.

There are many symptoms. These include:

- A weak, sluggish urinary stream, which may be particularly noticeable first thing in the morning; you may notice this as a thin stream, or you may not be able to urinate as high or as far as you used to.
- Difficulty in starting the flow of urine, known as hesitancy.
- A tendency to stop and start urinating, known as an intermittent flow.
- The feeling that you haven't quite emptied your bladder and that there is more to come.
- Straining to pass water.
- Incontinence – this is not an inevitable part of old age, it is a sign that there is something wrong.
- Dribbling of urine.
- Urinary retention.
- Pain or discomfort on passing water, known as dysuria.
- Blood in the urine, known as haematuria.
- The need to rush urgently to the toilet to pass water.
- Increasingly frequent need to pass water – perhaps as often as every two hours.

- Having to get up in the night to pass water (nocturia).
- The need to push or strain to pass water.
- Blood in the semen, known as haemospermia.

Self-help

Some men find that they are better able to empty their bladders efficiently when they urinate in a sitting or squatting position rather than standing up.

TAKING THE PROBLEM SERIOUSLY

The symptoms of an enlarged prostate must never be dismissed as an inevitable part of the ageing process. If a man does not seek medical help, there are two things that can happen.

Firstly, he may suddenly become totally incapable of passing urine. This is very painful and requires urgent treatment in hospital, whereby a tube (catheter) has to be passed into the bladder in order to drain off the excess urine.

When an enlarged prostate is not a problem

If the prostate is enlarged, as detected by a digital rectal examination, but there are no symptoms, there is no need for treatment. The size of the gland alone is no indication calling for treatment – still less for surgery. Intervention for benign enlargement should only be considered when the symptoms become a problem.

Secondly, the other thing that may happen is that the bladder can become so stretched that every time a man passes urine he does not quite empty it. The bladder expands very gradually, with the result that there is no pain and there may be no obvious symptoms for a while. Eventually, however, he will pass urine in a dribble, and he may notice that he is constantly wetting his underpants. He may even find that he is wetting the bed at night (known as enuresis), which is a distressing and embarrassing symptom. In extreme cases, the end result of this may be that there is so much back pressure on the kidneys that they eventually fail. This is a very serious condition, known as chronic retention of urine with renal failure.

THE RISKS

A benign enlarged prostate is not, in itself, a dangerous condition, but there are three main risks which may arise if the condition is not treated.

- Firstly, if the bladder is never completely emptied, there may be a build-up of stagnant urine in it. This can become a breeding ground for bacteria and can cause cystitis, which is an inflammation of the inner lining of the bladder. Treatment is by the administration of antibiotics.

- Secondly, the muscular walls of the bladder strengthen in an attempt to force urine through the narrowed urethra. As a result, the walls may become thickened and can then pinch the tubes that carry urine from the kidneys to the bladder, known as the ureters. Back pressure may cause acute pyelonephritis, which is an inflammation of the kidney, usually caused by bacterial infection, leading to symptoms such as high fever, chills and back pain. Treatment is usually by antibiotic drugs, which may need to be given by intravenous infusions.

- And finally, the muscles of the bladder may become weakened and no longer able to overcome the resistance to urine flow. They may then cease to function completely, which may be a sudden or a gradual process. A sudden failure to function may cause acute retention, which is very painful and requires emergency treatment. A gradual failure can lead to stress incontinence, causing a dribble of urine whenever a man affected coughs, sneezes or laughs. In an extreme case, if the condition remains untreated, the sufferer may eventually develop acute retention or even kidney failure.

THE INTERNATIONAL PROSTATE SYMPTOMS SCORE

The World Health Organization (WHO) recently devised a system, known as the International Prostate Symptoms Score. This enables you – and your doctor – to judge how severe your prostate symptoms are and how urgently – or if – you need treatment.

INTERNATIONAL PROSTATE SYMPTOMS SCORE						
	Not at all	Less than one time in five	Less than half the time	About half the time	More than half the time	Almost always
Over the past month: How often have you had the sensation of not completely emptying your bladder after urinating?	0	1	2	3	4	5
Needed to urinate again within two hours of finishing urinating?	0	1	2	3	4	5
Stopped and started again several times when urinating?	0	1	2	3	4	5
Found it difficult to postpone urinating?	0	1	2	3	4	5
Had to push or strain to start urinating?	0	1	2	3	4	5
Had to get up in the night to urinate?	0	1	2	3	4	5

How did you score?

- 0–8: your symptoms are very mild. You may not need any treatment but your symptoms will be closely monitored by your doctor. You may benefit from a change in diet or extracts of rye pollen.
- 9–17: your symptoms are moderate. Your doctor may prescribe a drug treatment, provided that your rectal examination and blood tests are normal.
- 17 and over: your symptoms are severe. Your doctor will probably refer you to a specialist for further tests and treatment.

WHAT TO DO

It is not uncommon for a man who is experiencing symptoms of an enlarged prostate to put off going to the doctor. He may do this because he has heard that the doctor will probably give him a rectal examination and he would rather avoid this. Or he may do it because he thinks that his symptoms are an inevitable part of growing old and that the doctor will not take them seriously. But he is wrong.

The doctor *will* take them seriously and, as I have already said, he should not delay. Treatment nowadays is both straightforward and effective, and it is sensible to have treatment before your disease progresses and you are at any risk.

Early screening may help prevent you developing problems in the future with your kidneys. Even more importantly, it may ensure that the still more serious but rare problem of prostate cancer is discovered early – and therefore treated early.

WHAT YOUR DOCTOR WILL DO

There are several things your doctor and/or a specialist, known as a urologist, may do to investigate an enlarged prostate, and to decide which treatment would be most appropriate.

These may include any or all of the following:

- Digital rectal examination (DRE).
- Blood tests.
- Urine tests.
- Ultrasound.
- CyStoscopy.
- Intravenous pyelogram (IVP).

Digital rectal examination (DRE)

The first investigation a doctor will probably do is a digital rectal examination. To do this, he will gently insert his gloved index finger into your rectum. He will use a water-based jelly as a lubricant. A rectal examination does not hurt, and you should not feel embarrassed – it's all in a day's work to a doctor.

The shape and size, as well as the texture and tenderness of the prostate can be felt in this way. If you have an enlarged prostate, the gland will feel just that – enlarged. It will also feel firm and smooth.

Blood tests

There are several blood tests that are likely to be done as part of the investigation of an enlarged prostate. These may be done to check for infection, to check how well your kidneys are working, and to eliminate prostate cancer (see Chapter 6).

Tests include:

- Full blood count, as a check for infection or anaemia.
- Urea and electrolytes, to see how well your kidneys are functioning.
- Prostate acid phosphatase (PAP), to check for prostate cancer.
- Prostate specific antigen (PSA), to check for prostate cancer.

Urine tests

Similarly, there are a number of urine tests that are likely to be done as part of the investigation of an enlarged prostate. These are done both to determine how badly your stream of urine is affected, and to check for infection.

Tests include:

- Urinary flow rate, using a urine-flow meter, which determines how badly your ability to urinate normally is affected. As you pass urine into a bottle, an electronic device measures both the total amount passed and the speed with which it is passed. This will reveal the extent of any obstruction to the flow.
- Mid stream urine (MSU), to check for any bacterial infection, which may indicate cystitis, and for any red blood or pus cells, as well as for any tiny threads of tissue shed from the kidney, known as casts.
- Urine dip stick test, to check for sugar and protein.

Ultrasound

This entails passing high-frequency sound waves through your body, which then bounce back off special tissue plates to produce an image on a screen. Ultrasound, or sonography, can reveal several things, including:

- The size of your prostate gland.
- Whether there is any residual urine (and, if so, how much), left in your bladder after urinating.
- The size of your kidneys.

Cystoscopy

This entails passing a narrow telescope, known as a cystoscope, through the penis and into the bladder. This procedure is done under general anaesthetic.

It enables the urethra and bladder to be viewed in detail, with the result that the degree of prostate obstruction can be assessed accurately.

Intravenous pyelogram (IVP)

This test entails injecting a radio-opaque form of iodine into a vein. The dye is then concentrated in the kidneys, and X-rays are taken of the urinary tract. These will therefore show any abnormalities. An IVP rules out the possibility that symptoms are due to urinary tract disease rather than to an enlarged prostate. It also reveals whether the bladder, ureters or kidneys have been damaged by back pressure from the enlargement.

TREATMENT OF AN ENLARGED PROSTATE

Exactly how the doctors decide to treat your enlarge prostate depends to a large extent on how severe your symptoms are (this is where the International Prostate Symptoms Score (see page 48) comes in useful and has a practical purpose; on whether your condition is threatening vital systems such as your kidneys; on how much it is affecting your lifestyle; and on your general state of health. Whatever you are offered, it is worth your while checking that you are being offered the most up-to-date treatment available. Treatments are being improved all the time, and it is a good idea to discuss this with your doctor or specialist. You should also voice any particular worries that you have. Don't worry about wasting your doctor's time – that's what he's there for and he should be happy to take the time and trouble to talk about your worries with you and to explain the situation.

Is it worth the risk?

You must talk to your doctor in some detail about possible treatments and their risks. Only you know how much your symptoms are affecting your life, and only you can decide what risks you are willing to take in order to get rid of them. Would it be worth a slight risk of impotence, for example, not to have to get up twice in the night to urinate? No one can answer this on your behalf – it's got to be your decision.

If symptoms are mild . . .

In this case, and if tests have ruled out any possibility of prostate cancer, doctors may adopt a 'wait-and-see' approach. Symptoms may not get any worse, and a modification to diet, along with extracts of rye pollen, may help (see Naturopathy, Chapter 9).

If symptoms are moderate . . .

In this case, a doctor may decide on a drug approach, which may help relieve symptoms. Possible drugs include:

- Alpha-blocker drugs, such as indoramin, prazosin and terazosin. These are the most commonly used form of drug treatment. They relax the nervous system and inhibit contractions in the prostate and urethra. In this way, they ease symptoms rather than counteracting the obstruction completely.

- Antispasmodic drugs, such as flavoxate, oxybutinin and propantheline, which reduce irritation of the bladder.

- 5-alpha-reductase inhibitors, such as finasteride, which prevent the hormone testosterone from being converted into dihydrotestosterone, which is known to cause an enlarged prostate. These drugs shrink the gland and may slightly improve the flow of urine.

If symptoms are severe . . .

Symptoms may be so severe that the urethra is blocked off completely, with the result that the sufferer is unable to pass urine. This is a very painful condition and requires immediate hospitalisation.

The recommended treatment in this case will probably be catheterisation, which entails inserting a flexible tube, or catheter, into the bladder under local anaesthetic to drain trapped urine. This will usually bring instant and welcome relief and, as such, is a valuable treatment.

It is not, however, considered to be an acceptable long-term solution by most men, who regard it only as a temporary measure until something permanent can be done. The long-term solution is usually surgery, in the form of a prostatectomy (see below).

If, however, surgery is considered to be too dangerous – usually because of ill health or advanced age – a catheter may be kept in place permanently. It will continue to provide drainage into a special bag that is worn attached to the leg.

Surgery

For many men, the only acceptable long-term solution is surgery. This entails the removal of either part, or all of, the prostate gland.

Most doctors advise an early operation, because the risk is much increased if the kidneys are already damaged. If surgery is performed when symptoms first become a serious nuisance, the results are nearly always very good.

The removal of part of the prostate is done by a procedure known as transurethral prostatectomy (TURP), in which prostate tissue is cut away using an electrically-heated wire loop inserted through the urethra. The entire prostate gland is removed in an operation known as a prostatectomy.

The more common of the two operations is TURP, though an open prostatectomy is sometimes chosen in preference to TURP. The reasons for this include the following:

- If the prostate is very much enlarged.

- If a tumour is suspected, which might be cured through the removal of the entire prostate.

- If a man also has large bladder stones, which also need to be removed.

- If a man has bad arthritis in the hips, which cannot therefore be placed up in stirrups, as this is needed for TURP.

Both transurethral prostatectomy and open prostatectomy are described in detail in Chapter 7.

Treatment by stent

A man who is too ill to withstand a major operation may have a stent implant put in place, This is a short, stiff tube that is placed in the urethra at the point at which it passes through the prostate gland. It holds the urethral walls open in spite of pressure from an enlarged gland. An advantage of this procedure is that a stent is simple to put in position and it can be done to a man who is not well enough to have a prostatectomy.

There are two types of stent: a permanent mesh type, which is left in position permanently and the skin of the urethra eventually grows over it; and a temporary spiral type, which can easily be removed but which has the disadvantage that it is prone to bacterial infection and that it can become dislodged.

Other possibilities

Medical advances have come up with several new procedures, some of which are still at the clinical trial stage. Research continues in this field, and the outlook for further advances in the treatment of this debilitating condition is good, though as yet most of these procedures are still a long way out of mainstream medical practice.

New procedures include:

- TULIP (Transurethral, ultrasound guided, laser-induced prostatectomy), which entails using a laser to cut away prostate tissue.

- Microwave hyperthermia, which involves inserting a microwave coil within a catheter into the urethra and heating it to a temperature of $45°C$ ($113°F$). The treatment must be done twice a week for three to five weeks. Each treatment takes between 30 and 60 minutes. There is no need for any anaesthetic and the procedure can be done as an out-patient. As yet, there have been no large-scale or long-term studies.

- Transrectal hyperthermia, which is another heat-shrinking procedure, introducing a probe into the rectum. This heats the prostate to a temperature of $43°C$ ($109°F$) using microwaves.

The procedure is usually repeated six times, and lasts one hour each time. During the treatment period, the patient can lead a normal life, suffering no more than slight discomfort each time.

- TUNA: Transurethral needle ablation, which means needles are inserted into the prostate, under local anaesthetic, to allow greater precision and higher temperatures during heat-shrinking procedures.

- Sonoblate, which is another heat-shrinking procedure, this time involving ultrasound waves via the rectum.

- Cryotherapy, which entails inserting a cryoprobe into the penis and freezing the prostate.

- Dilatation of the prostate with the use of balloons.

6 Cancer of the Prostate

Cancer of the prostate, or adenocarcinoma of the prostate, as it is technically called, is a malignant growth occurring in the prostate gland. It is an alarmingly common problem, though most men would probably be surprised to learn this. They will have heard of it – famous sufferers have included Frank Zappa, Roger Moore, macho Gulf War hero 'Stormin'' Norman Schwartzkopf and President François Mitterand – but they are unlikely to realise just how common it is.

This is surprising because it is, in fact, the most common type of cancer in men in Britain. It is also the second most common cause of death from cancer in men, after lung cancer. According to the Imperial Cancer Research Fund, it kills nearly 10,000 men a year in Britain, which is four times as many men as women who die from cervical cancer. Some 14,000 new cases of prostate cancer are diagnosed each year in Britain. But ask the average man in the street where his prostate gland is, and the chances are he won't be able to tell you.

A DISEASE OF OLD AGE

Prostate cancer most often occurs in the elderly, though it does sometimes develop in middle age. More precisely, it is most common in men over the age of 55, and becomes increasingly common as a man gets older. Nearly all deaths caused by prostate cancer occur in men over the age of 65, while half of all cases occur in men over the age of 75. Peak age is between 70 and 80.

People worry that cancer of the prostate seems to be on the

increase, but this is not necessarily as sinister a prospect as may at first appear. More screening is being done, which is bound to reveal an increase in figures. And it is, in any case, more characteristically a disease of old age than any other cancer. As there are more and more elderly people in the population today, it is not surprising that prostate cancer has become correspondingly more common too.

SURVIVAL RATES

The question in the mind of any man who is reading this will probably be: If I get prostate cancer, what are my chances of survival?

The answer to this vexed question is not a simple or an obvious one. This is because it depends on so many things:

- How old you are.
- The state of your overall health, prostate apart.
- At what stage the cancer was discovered.

In a man over the age of 70, the survival rate is about 50 per cent. It is higher in a younger man – the younger he is, the greater his chances of survival. His chances are also higher if the cancer was detected early on in its growth.

WHAT CAUSES IT?

The exact cause of prostate cancer remains a mystery, though the male hormone testosterone appears to have some involvement. Quite what that is, though, is not certain.

Certain risk factors have, however, been identified. Firstly, and like a great many cancers, cancer of the prostate is known to run in families. If a close relative – say, a brother or father – has cancer of the prostate, a man's risk of developing the disease seems to be nearly three times greater than that of a man who does not have any family history of the disease. If a man has more than one relative with prostate cancer – say, a grandfather or uncle as well as a brother or father – his chances of developing the disease are as many as six times greater than that of a man who does not have any family history of the disease.

There do, however, seem to be other factors involved. Diet is one of these. The typical UK diet, for example – which is usually low in green vegetables, fruit and pulses and high in animal fats in the form of meat and dairy products – may well be a contributing factor.

According to the Cancer Research Campaign, black American men have the highest incidence of prostate cancer, with some 50 per cent more cases than in the US white male population. This is probably because they have a higher than usual level of testosterone.

The number of sexual partners a man has had may have a link with the development of prostate cancer, though this has not been proved. In particular, the wart virus (human papilloma virus), which is usually sexually transmitted, may increase a man's chances of developing cancer of the prostate, in much the same way as it predisposes a woman to developing cancer of the cervix.

SYMPTOMS

Very often there are, unfortunately, no early signs of prostate cancer, which makes its early detection very difficult. The great majority – up to 90 per cent – of cancers begin on the outside of the prostate, which means that they do not usually obstruct urinary flow in the early stages of the disease, and can therefore go unnoticed for some time.

And they can remain undetected for some time because prostate cancer is very slow in spreading. It may be as long as four years before the cancer has doubled in size, and this, too, makes its early diagnosis very difficult unless people have routine screening for the disease.

In its later stages, however, prostate cancer has similar symptoms to those of an enlarged prostate. It is not unusual, in fact, for a man who is being investigated for an enlarged prostate to have cancer diagnosed. That is not intended to be alarmist, however, and any man who is being investigated for an enlarged prostate should not panic. An enlarged prostate is ten times more common than prostate cancer, so the odds are greatly in your favour – it's just that the two conditions do have similar symptoms. As has already been discussed (see Chapter 5), the symptoms of an enlarged prostate are:

- A weak, sluggish urinary stream, which may be particularly noticeable first thing in the morning; you may notice this as a thin stream, or you may not be able to urinate as high or as far as you used to.
- Difficulty in starting the flow of urine, known as hesitancy.
- A tendency to stop and start urinating, known as an intermittent flow.
- The feeling that you haven't quite emptied your bladder and that there is more to come.
- Straining to pass water.
- Incontinence – this is not an inevitable part of old age, it is a sign that there is something wrong.
- Dribbling of urine.
- Urinary retention.
- Pain or discomfort on passing water, known as dysuria.
- Blood in the urine, known as haematuria.
- The need to rush urgently to the toilet to pass water.
- Increasingly frequent need to pass water – perhaps as often as every two hours.
- Having to get up in the night to pass water.
- The need to push or strain to pass water.
- Blood in the semen, known as haemospermia.

There may, however, be no urinary symptoms at all. The first sign of the disease may be from secondary growths, or metastases, of the cancer, which are most commonly in the bones. Prostate cancer has a tendency to spread to the bones, and this happens in a high proportion of cases.

Symptoms of cancer of the bone:

- Pain in the bone, which is often worse at night.
- Bone tenderness.
- Brittle bones, which may suddenly break without any injury.
- Fatigue.
- Loss of appetite.
- Weight loss.
- Anaemia.

Bone cancer

A malignant growth in the bone can be primary, in which case it originates in the bone itself; or secondary, in which case it has spread from cancer elsewhere in the body. Secondary bone cancer, or metastatic cancer, is more common than primary bone cancer, and prostate cancer is one of the cancers that spreads readily to the bone.

Bone metastases occur most commonly in:

- The spine.
- The ribs.
- The hips.
- The pelvis.
- The upper legs.
- The skull.

Secondary bone cancers from the prostate often respond well to hormonal treatment, including oestrogen or hypothalamic hormones. Sometimes the most effective treatment may be by removal of the testes, or adrenal glands. The administration of a radioactive isotope such as Metastron is used to relieve pain from bone cancer.

DIAGNOSIS

In most cases, cancer develops in the outer part of the prostate gland, where it can be felt as a small, hard lump. Cancer of the prostate is usually diagnosed during a digital rectal examination. If the prostate gland is cancerous, it will feel hard and knobbly.

The diagnosis may be confirmed in a number of ways. These include:

- Ultrasound scanning of the prostate gland, whereby a probe is inserted into the rectum and detects tumours as abnormal echoes of sound.

- Urography, also known as pyelography, which is a procedure for obtaining X-rays of the urinary tract, which involves introducing a radio-opaque medium into the bloodstream.

- Prostatic biopsy, whereby a sample of tissue is removed for examination under the microscope. This is probably the most reliable way of determining whether a growth is benign or malignant. A small sample of tissue is removed from the tumour under local anaesthetic with a fine needle.

- A blood test, which measures the level of the protein prostate specific antigen (PSA). This is a protein manufactured only by prostate cells. If the blood test reveals a normal level of PSA – that is less than 4 ng/ml – there is very little chance of prostate cancer. If it reveals a level of PSA that is between 4 and 10 ng/ml, there is a 20 per cent chance of prostate cancer. And, if the level is above 10 ng/ml, there is a 60 per cent chance of prostate cancer. Unfortunately, small cancerous growths are often not revealed by this test, which can give both false negatives and false positives. It has a useful role, though, in conjunction with other tests, such an ultrasound scan or a CT scan.

- A blood test for anaemia.

- A blood test to check kidney function.

- A blood test which measures the level of prostatic acid phosphatase (PAP). This is a blood enzyme which indicates whether prostate cancer has spread to form secondary bone cancer.

- A bone scan, which will enable doctors to ascertain how far the cancer has spread into the bones. This is only done once prostate cancer has been confirmed.

- A CT scan, which uses an electronic X-ray detector to build up a 3-D picture of your body in cross-section, as if a slice had been taken from it. This will enable doctors to see how far the cancer has spread into surrounding tissues.

- A lymphangiogram, which involves injecting a special dye into the lymph vessels and monitoring their progress. This enables doctors to see if cancer has reached the pelvic lymph nodes.

If your doctor finds a lump . . .

If your doctor finds a lump during a digital rectal examination, you should try not to worry. This is easier said than done but it is reassuring to know that most lumps are not in fact cancerous. It is estimated that in around half of the cases sent for further tests, no trace of cancer is found. A lump may be due to a bladder stone or it may have some other benign cause.

ROUTINE SCREENING

How early prostate cancer is detected depends, to a large extent on where you live. In the UK, routine screening does not, on the whole, happen as a matter of course, which means that few cancers – substantially under half – are caught in the early stages. In the US, on the other hand, most men are screened annually, with the result that rather more cancers of the prostate – well over half – are picked up in the early stages.

Routine screening can be done in several ways. These include:

- A blood test measuring the level of the protein prostate specific antigen (PSA) (see page 62).

- A digital rectal examination, whereby the doctor feels the prostate through the rectum to see whether it has become hard and knobbly.
- Transrectal ultrasound (TRUS) of the prostate gland.

The value of screening

This is a highly controversial question, as there is some doubt as to whether or not the early treatment of prostate cancer actually increases the chances of a cure.

Prostate cancer tends to be a cancer associated with old age and cancers tend to grow more slowly as you get older. Because prostate cancer is so slow-growing, there are many elderly men suffering from this disease who never actually die of it. Many of them die of something else before their cancer becomes life-threatening.

Research into the value of early intervention continues. The Medical Research Council in the UK is currently researching this very question, with the help of urologists throughout the country.

The earlier the better?

It is sometimes possible to detect prostate cancer early enough to treat it successfully, but this is not always the case and it is therefore not certain that the earlier the cancer is detected the better the chances of a cure. Cancer of the prostate is not always consistent in its response to treatment.

Sometimes it spreads rapidly and can cause death in a very short time – even as short a time as a year from diagnosis. Sometimes, on the other hand – more often than not, in fact – it progresses very slowly and can be kept under control for a long time. And sometimes it causes no symptoms at all, and it is only known that the patient suffered from it when a post-mortem is done after the patient has died from some other, quite different cause.

National screening programmes for prostate cancer would be very expensive. They are unlikely to be set up in Britain until there are better ways of identifying which cases would benefit most from treatment.

In the meantime, and until the results become available, many doctors are particularly keen on annual prostate specific antigen (PSA) blood tests to detect early prostate trouble. This is not always available on the NHS.

TREATMENT

Prostate cancer may be treated in a number of ways. Treatment varies widely from country to country, even from one urologist to another. This is an unpredictable disease, and there is plenty of room for argument as to which treatment is likely to be better.

Treatment varies, in any case, according to how early the cancer has been discovered and on how far it has spread. If it has spread beyond the prostate gland, the specialist is likely to decide that it is better to aim treatment at controlling the condition rather than attempting to cure it.

Treatment also depends on the patient – how old he is, and how well he is. In some cases, the side-effects of treatment may outweigh the benefits, particularly as about half of all men aged between 70 and 80 develop prostate cancer which never spreads beyond the prostate and which never becomes life-threatening. In these cases, the best treatment of all is no treatment.

However, if treatment is decided on, it may be done in the following ways:

- The surgical removal of the prostate, which is known as prostatectomy (see Chapter 7).
- Radiotherapy, which involves passing radiation through the diseased tissue and so destroying the abnormal cells or slowing down their development. This is usually given externally and done every day for several weeks. Radiotherapy is particularly

recommended for early prostate cancers, when it has the same success rate as surgery, and for particularly large tumours within the prostate. Side-effects include diarrhoea, rectal discomfort, painful urination and blood in the urine. It can also cause impotence as a result of the effects of radiation on the blood vessels supplying the penis.

If the cancer has spread to other parts of the body, patients may benefit from reducing their level of the male hormone testosterone. This can be done by:

- Orchidectomy, which is the surgical removal of the testes. Surgical castration is obviously a drastic measure, which can be very traumatic for the patient. The testes may be replaced by egg-shaped implants which are inserted in the scrotum to look and feel as much like the real thing as possible. Orchidectomy has several unpleasant side-effects, such as hot flushes (a bit like those experienced by menopausal women), impotence and loss of libido.

- The administration of oestrogen drugs, which have the unfortunate side-effects of breast enlargement and the reduction of libido.

- The administration of anti-androgens, which block the action of testosterone and thereby inhibit further growth and spread of cancer.

- The administration of drugs that block the release of the pituitary hormone, which, in turn, controls the release of testosterone. Known as medical castration, this has the inevitable side-effects of hot flushes, impotence and a low sex drive, but is as effective as surgical castration and not as traumatic, either physically or psychologically. The other great advantage that medical castration has over surgical castration is that it can be reversed. Drug therapy has improved considerably in recent years, and injections these days may only need to be given every 12 weeks.

- The administration of an anti-androgen in combination with medical castration.

- Radiotherapy, which shrinks the prostate gland or relieves the pain of secondary bone cancer, if it exists.

OUTLOOK

Overall survival with prostate cancer at five years is 20 per cent. If the cancer is diagnosed at an early stage, the outlook is very good. According to the Cancer Research Fund, as many as 43 per cent live for five years or more following diagnosis. If, on the other hand, the cancer has already spread beyond the prostate gland and fails to respond to hormone treatment, the outlook is poor.

Taking a positive approach

It is well worth bearing in mind that those patients suffering from cancer – any kind of cancer – who are able to develop and maintain a positive approach to their illness usually cope better with it, and actually fare better, than those patients who get very depressed and negative in their outlook. Some doctors actually believe that a positive approach helps to reinforce the body's natural defence mechanisms and immune responses, and may therefore enable a person to fight an illness – and to win.

Eating for a healthy prostate

There is a much lower incidence of prostate cancer in some parts of the world, which indicates that certain diets may well protect against prostate cancer, while others may actually trigger it. In particular, men in China and Japan are known to have a lower incidence of prostatitis, enlarged prostate and prostate cancer than their counterparts in the West. If Eastern men move to the West, their incidence rate rises again, indicating that they do not have an inherited protection and suggesting that it is their way of life and eating habits while living in the East that offer them protection. The traditional Eastern diet is low in fat, consisting of soya products, fish, grains and vegetables, particularly yellow, orange, red and green vegetables, and those from the cabbage and turnip families (see also DIET, Chapter 10).

7 Prostatectomy

Prostatectomy is an operation to remove part or all of the prostate gland. It always necessitates a stay in hospital.

Surgery is still the treatment of first choice in the great majority of cases of an enlarged prostate. It is, in fact, a very common operation, with some 40,000 operations being performed each year in Britain. In the US, an astonishing 400,000 operations are performed each year. Prostatectomy is, in fact, the fourth most common operation performed on men in the US, with the competition for top place coming from cataract removal, hernia repair, and gall-bladder operations. Estimated total cost spent on prostate removal in the US is over 1,500 million dollars.

Prostatectomy is usually performed for one of two reasons. These are:

• When the gland is so enlarged that it obstructs the flow of urine.

• When prostate cancer had been diagnosed and surgery is considered to be the best option.

Success rates

The chances of success of a prostatectomy, in terms of the removal of obstruction and the resulting relief of symptoms, are very high indeed. Looked at from the point of view of doctors, with reference to the removal of the urethral obstruction, the success rate is an amazing 90 per cent. And looked at from the point of view of patients, with reference to the relief of their symptoms, the success rate is 80 per cent.

Getting the timing right

It is important, if you are having a prostatectomy, to get the timing right. Have it too early, when your symptoms are still mild, and you have a lower than average chance of relieving symptoms and a higher than average chance of having to have a repeat operation later. A repeat operation is particularly likely if you have your first operation before you are 60, as did Ronald Reagan. If, on the other hand, you have it too late, your prostate problem may by then be so severe that it will have affected your general health so much that doctors consider it too risky for you to have the operation at all, or your bladder may never be able to recover its former strength.

It is often not possible for doctors to predict how quickly, or how slowly, a man's condition is likely to deteriorate. A man with moderate symptoms may not get any worse for many years, while another man with slight symptoms may suddenly find he needs emergency treatment.

Equally, it is often impossible for a doctor to predict what effect an operation will have. It will probably bring dramatic and substantial improvement, but it may not.

APPROACHING THE PROSTATE GLAND

The prostate gland is situated in a very inaccessible part of the body. This means that an operation to remove it can be difficult.

The other possible problem is that, because it is close to the opening of the bladder, there is a danger of damaging the delicate muscles that prevent urine from leaking between acts of urination.

There are two ways of approaching the prostate gland. It can be approached:

- Via the bladder, in an operation known as transurethral prostatectomy (TURP).

- Via the abdomen, in an operation known as open prostatectomy.

The end result of the two operations are basically similar, but an open prostatectomy is a more major operation than a TURP, so you can expect to feel worse for a longer period of time than after a TURP.

TRANSURETHRAL PROSTATECTOMY (TURP)

This is the removal of the prostate gland by way of the urethra, without making any incision through the skin. TURP is by far the more common method of surgery. It is used in as many as 90 per cent of patients undergoing a prostatectomy.

The advantage of TURP is that the patient has no surgical incision. This means that there is no need for general anaesthetic, it is a much less invasive and safer procedure, and the patient suffers less discomfort or pain after the operation. TURP is a far less traumatic procedure altogether for the body, and patients therefore make a much quicker recovery. It necessitates a hospital stay for about four or five days.

How it is done

The man's legs are placed in padded stirrups, rather like what sometimes happens when a woman is having a baby, and the genitalia are washed with detergent and water. A fine, telescope-like type of cystoscope, or bladder viewing tube, known as a resectoscope, is then passed up the penis into the bladder. This instrument, which has a fibre-optic light and a lens system, enables the surgeon to look at the urethra and at the obstructing part of the prostate. It also has a special cautery (searing) device with a heated wire loop on the end, which is attached to an electric current. Each time the wire loop moves through the tissue, little pieces of tissue in the prostate gland are chipped away, in much the same way as an apple is cored.

The new growth in the prostate occurs in the centre, so the operation removes this tissue, working back outwards to the original

71

prostate tissue, in much the same way as you insert a knife into the core of an apple and remove the flesh from the inside back towards the skin until all the core has been removed. The TURP procedure takes about an hour.

The pieces of prostatic tissue are washed out through the resectoscope, and bleeding vessels are cauterised by an electrode, which is passed up the tube. The resectoscope is then removed, and a catheter is passed up the urethra into the bladder, in order to drain urine and allow blood to be removed. This is left in place for several days.

It may take some time for symptoms to settle down after a TURP, though they usually do settle down, sometimes with the aid of medication. In a few cases – around 15 per cent – the prostate gland continues to enlarge after surgery, and symptoms eventually recur so that another TURP is needed only a few years – usually around eight years – later.

This happened to Ronald Reagan, who had a second prostate operation during his first term as President. You may remember seeing him on the television as he went into Washington's Bethesda Naval Hospital accompanied by his wife Nancy, with the words, "We've been here before!".

Modern equipment

It wasn't until sometime between the two World Wars that prostate surgery through the urethra became a practical procedure. Even then, before the invention of the fibre-optic light source and the lens system used for this operation, transurethral prostatic surgery used to be considered one of the most difficult operations for the surgeon to learn. Modern equipment has succeeded in revolutionising the operation, which is now relatively simply, quick and straightforward.

Testing for cancer

In this way, the surgeon is able to collect some of the tissue for investigation under a microscope that will (in most cases) rule out prostate cancer. You will be told a day or two after the operation what the result is. Unsuspected cancer is found in about 5 per cent of patients undergoing a TURP.

Even if cancer cells are discovered, this is not necessarily a cause for any great alarm. The presence of cancer cells in the prostate gland is quite common in older men, and your surgeon should give you some idea of the extent of the cancer found. You may be given some radiation or chemotherapy straight away, or you may be referred for further scanning or other tests to establish whether the cancer has spread beyond the prostate. If your urologist did not detect the presence of cancer during a rectal examination, this is unlikely.

OPEN PROSTATECTOMY

This operation is performed on only 10 per cent of men undergoing a prostatectomy. It is usually reserved for the removal of a particularly large prostate gland. It is also done where an operation on the bladder – say, the removal of bladder stones, for example – has to be done at the same time.

An open prostatectomy is performed under general anaesthetic. It usually means staying in hospital for seven to ten days.

How it is done

The operation entails making a cut across the lower abdomen, to expose the bladder and prostate. The prostate gland is then approached via the space between the back of the pubic bone and the bladder.

The first open prostate operations were performed towards the end of the nineteenth century, both in England and in the US. These early operations carried a high mortality rate and were therefore not performed very often, nor in many hospitals. At the turn of the twentieth century, there were still only two common treatments for severe prostate enlargement – catheterisation and, still more puzzlingly, vasectomy, which seems to have been a misguided procedure for this condition.

The first really successful open operations, which were not only effective but also safe – were performed by Sir Peter Freyer of St Peter's Hospital in Covent Garden. This was hailed as the moment when 'a dangerous surgical adventure became a routine operation'. Open prostate operations became common in the years between the two World Wars, but there was still a relatively high mortality rate of between 5 and 15 per cent.

The surgeon cuts open the capsule containing the prostate gland, which is then 'shelled out' from the inside. Bleeding vessels are cauterised, and a catheter is passed up the urethra to drain urine from the bladder. A tube is also inserted beside the empty capsule to drain fluid and to prevent blood clots forming. The abdomen is then sewn up and both catheter and tube are usually left in place for approximately five to seven days after the operation, and are then removed as long as there is no residual bleeding.

AFTER-EFFECTS

Bleeding may be so severe after the operation that blood transfusions are required. Any blood clots that form within the bladder as a result of the operation can usually be washed out through the catheter, which is why it is left in place for several days afterwards.

When the catheter is removed, patients often notice that their urination has been affected. It is usually more frequent than normal, and may also be painful. Some patients even suffer from a mild form of incontinence for anything up to a few weeks afterwards. It is important for patients to drink large amounts of fluid in order to help wash out any remaining blood in the urine.

Most patients resume all their normal activities after several weeks following the operation. They are likely to recover more slowly after an open prostatectomy than they are after a TURP.

Serious complications

Most men have a straightforward recovery after a prostatectomy (see Chapter 7). A few men, however – about one in five men – may suffer from serious complications after an open prostatectomy of the kind that can happen after any operation. These include infection, or embolism in the lung. A few others may develop minor problems such as urinary infections, or more serious ones such as a stricture, or a narrowing of the urethra, which is usually caused by scarring. This may cause worse obstructive symptoms than those caused by the original prostate problem and will necessitate further surgery in order to put it right.

The most serious complication is death. This is rare after prostatectomy, though general anaesthesia and surgery always carry some degree of risk. You should be aware of this before deciding on surgery, though you should not dwell on it.

RESUMING SEXUAL ACTIVITIES

A man's sex life should not be affected after a prostatectomy. Uncommonly, however, some men do experience sexual problems – notably a decrease in sexual sensation and a change in the intensity of their orgasms. This may, in turn, have an adverse effect on their sex drive.

A prostatectomy may cause some damage to the nerve supply to the penis, particularly with an open prostatectomy. Some men may therefore lose their potency after the operation, though this is rare.

Sterility

A much more common after-effect of a prostatectomy is for a man to become sterile. This is because semen is expelled backwards into the bladder at orgasm, as opposed to being ejaculated from the penis. This condition is known as retrograde ejaculation. It happens because it is usually impossible to remove the obstructing part of the prostate gland without also removing the muscle that contracts and blocks off the neck of the bladder during intercourse, and normally ensures that a man ejaculates semen when he has an orgasm and not urine.

According to evidence given by urologists on both sides of the Atlantic, it is estimated that retrograde ejaculation affects between 30 and 90 per cent of men who have had a prostatectomy. Retrograde ejaculation does not usually cause a problem, and sperm will be voided, quite simply, the next time he urinates and empties his bladder. The presence of sperm in the bladder is in no way harmful, and it does not harm the penis, the bladder, or you. Most men report that this does have an effect on the sensation of orgasm.

The only problem occurs if a man wants to have children in the future, as he will now be subfertile. It used to be thought that most men undergoing prostatectomy are of an age when they will probably have completed their families and are unlikely to wish to have any more children. In this case, sterility would obviously not be a great problem. But nowadays, with an increasing divorce rate and more and more men marrying second (and often younger) wives, this assumption can no longer be made.

If a man wants to have children, or thinks he might want to do so in the future, it is possible to aspirate sperm from the bladder and use this for artificial insemination. It is recommended, however, that he pre-empts this possibility by having sperm frozen and stored in a sperm bank *before* he undergoes the operation.

This involves producing sperm by masturbation, and having it deep-frozen and stored. Success is not guaranteed, though it does give you a pretty good chance. It is rarely available on the National Health Service, and it is worth comparing the prices of several different services as they can vary a lot. Your best bet is to try hospitals that have a reputation for infertility work. You can also obtain a list of centres registered with the Human Fertilisation and Embryology Authority. The British Pregnancy Advisory Service and Marie Stopes both offer this as part of their service.

Contraception

You may have looked upon the sterility associated with prostatectomy as a good thing – no more need to worry about contraception. But although prostatectomy often causes sterility in a man, it offers no guarantees. Between 5 and 10 per cent of men are, in fact, still fertile afterwards – which may be good news for some of you but bad news for others. If you want a reliable and permanent method of contraception, you should discuss the possibility of having a vasectomy with your surgeon, as this can easily be done at the same time.

ADVANCES IN SURGERY

Surgery has come a long way in recent years and there are new advances all the time, which make the future a brighter and more hopeful place. The use of lasers, which are thought by many to be the most accurate and efficient of surgical tools, in prostate surgery is still at an experimental stage.

Even more amazingly, prostate surgery can now be done by a robotic surgeon – more quickly, accurately, precisely and efficiently than could be done by any human being. The TURP operation is different from most other operations in that it involves a lengthy series of repetitive movements to cut away the enlarged tissues. Robots are particularly good at performing repetitive tasks with great accuracy. The robot also has an impressive understanding of three dimensions, which is something that surgeons are not always so good at, and often have to go back to the initial starting position during an operation to reorientate themselves. Should you worry about the idea of being in the 'hands' of a robot, rest assured: the surgeon can watch what is happening on a visual display unit and is thus able to monitor proceedings throughout the operation.

The possibility of robotic surgery has tremendous implications for the patient, not least of which is that it takes less time, which means that more patients can be treated on one patient list, and therefore dramatically shortens the ever-increasing waiting-list for operations. It gives every man hope for the future.

WAITING FOR SURGERY

There are thousands of men currently awaiting prostate surgery in Britain. Many of them will already have been waiting for longer than six months, and some for over a year.

Judging by the latest statistics, the chances are high that you'll spend considerable time on a hospital waiting-list. Talk to your consultant, who will have a pretty good idea of how many patients he has on his waiting-list, and where your case comes on his list in order of urgency.

In the meantime, you might like to try one of the self-help measures outlined in Chapter 10.

If you're losing patience, there are various ways in which you might be able to move further up the queue. Ask your doctor to write to your consultant about any circumstances that might help your case – if your condition is making it difficult for you to do your job, for example, or if your personal circumstances mean that you are finding it very difficult to cope with life before your operation, or –

perhaps most importantly – if your condition has worsened since your consultant last saw you.

You may find it beneficial to move to a different hospital, where the waiting-list is shorter. Your doctor should be able to help you, or you can call the College of Health's Helpline (0181-983 1133, Monday to Friday 10 a.m. to 4 p.m.), which keeps all the latest information on waiting-lists.

The other possibility, if you can afford it or if you are covered by private medical health insurance, is to go private. Prices vary enormously, so do a bit of research and find out how much it costs where, and what is included in the price.

Prostate surgery

Prostate surgery is probably the most common urological operation performed in this country. It costs the National Health Service an untold fortune. It is responsible for filling thousands of hospital beds throughout the country, and several thousands more are waiting for their operations.

---

8 Recovery from Prostate Surgery

Whatever anyone tells you, a prostatectomy is a major operation and you need to allow yourself sufficient time to recover from it. Men are notoriously impatient, especially if they have to go back to work, but you must accept that you will probably have to slow down for a while.

Don't expect miracles, and don't be too hard on yourself. You may not have had a leg amputated, but you have nevertheless had a major operation and you must make allowances for this. You must not expect too much of yourself during your recovery period in order to give yourself the best chance to get better as quickly as possible. Any impatience may, in the long run, only make matters worse and set you back on your road to recovery.

Exactly how long it takes you to get yourself back to a state of good health depends to a large extent on how fit you were before you had the operation. It also depends on how large your prostate gland was, and on whether or not there were any complications as a result of surgery.

Remember that old cliché about time being the great healer? It may not be very original but, like a lot of clichés, it's true. So grit your teeth and take things easy for a while. It may take as long as three months before you feel completely well again, but once you do, you'll be utterly convinced that it was worth every minute!

Your bladder

In the first few weeks after your operation, don't be surprised if your symptoms do not seem any better than before. They may even seem worse. This doesn't mean that the operation hasn't been a success – only that you haven't healed yet.

It can take anything up to about six weeks for the cut surface inside the prostate to heal over completely. Expecting everything to work perfectly before this happens is unrealistic. Until then, you will have to be prepared to make allowances.

Even when your urinary system returns to a state of good health, do not be surprised if you have problems getting used to this. You've probably spent a long time – years maybe – getting used to having to empty your bladder all too frequently, and it may take a long time – several weeks, probably, or even months – before you succeed in unlearning those habits. Be patient and you will gradually build up confidence in your bladder again until you are able to forget about it completely.

Medication

You will probably still be taking a course of antibiotics when you leave hospital. You must be disciplined about taking these. Remember to finish the course, and don't just stop taking the pills as soon as you feel better. This could set you back a long way and allow any leftover bacteria to multiply and mount another attack just when you're least expecting it and you're congratulating yourself on getting better.

AFTER AN OPEN PROSTATECTOMY

If you've had an open prostatectomy, you will have stitches in your abdomen and you will have been given strict instructions on what you can and can't do. You will be tired after your general anaesthetic and you will need to look after your wound. A district nurse will probably come to your house every other day to change the dressing, and she will take the stitches out when necessary.

You will have been told what movements you can make to avoid putting too great a strain on both the scar and the surrounding muscles. You should also:

- Avoid carrying anything at all heavy – even a full kettle may be too heavy, so fill it only half full.
- Get out of your chair cautiously and gently by wriggling your way to the edge of the chair before getting up.
- Build up slowly to normal activities.
- Use your common sense at all times and don't attempt to do too much.
- STOP immediately if you suspect you are doing too much.

Once you've had the stitches removed

Even when you've had the stitches removed, you will still need to be careful. It takes a good six weeks for the wound to heal itself, and several months before the abdominal muscles get back to their full strength.

AFTER A TRANSURETHRAL PROSTATECTOMY (TURP)

If, on the other hand, you've had the more common transurethral prostatectomy (TURP), you won't have any visible signs of your operation, like a scar, and it's all too easy to forget that you've actually had an operation at all. But you have, and you mustn't forget it.

Any operation puts a great physical strain on the body and, as a result, takes a surprisingly long time for you to get over. In hospital, you will have spent most of your time sitting or lying in bed. You probably won't have done anything more strenuous than reading or watching television. As soon as you get home, the temptation will be to resume all your favourite occupations – going for a walk in the park, perhaps, or doing a bit of gardening. But it is not a good idea to get back into the swing of things too soon. This should be a slow and gradual process, and you must be careful not to push yourself too far, or to do more than you can genuinely cope with.

In the meantime, make sure that you get plenty of rest. Get up late, have a rest whenever you feel you need one, and go to bed early. Whenever you are sitting, remember that a firm seat is more comfortable than a soft one that can press upwards between the buttocks.

The problem is obviously greater for people who live alone and who are looking after themselves. But even where this is the case – perhaps even more so, in fact, because you can't risk driving yourself so hard that you make yourself ill – you must restrict yourself at first to doing the essentials. You'll obviously need to do the cooking and washing, but most other things can wait.

There is absolutely no shame in spoiling yourself at a time like this. Your priority is to get well, and everything else comes second to that.

HAVING PLENTY TO DRINK

Whatever type of prostatectomy you've just had, it is a good idea to keep up your intake of fluids – preferably as much as 3.4 litres/6 pints a day. This may sound a lot, particularly if you've been used to limiting your fluid intake because of your need to urinate so frequently, but it is important because it helps your bladder to build up its strength and to return to normal.

Drinking plenty of liquid also helps to ward off infection and to soothe any bladder irritation. It helps, too, to wash out any little pieces of scab and blood from the cut surface inside the prostate, which is likely to happen for the first six to eight weeks after the operation. Although you may notice signs of blood in your urine at first, you should not feel any pain.

Contact your doctor if:

- You feel pain.
- You notice any large amounts of deep red blood in your urine.
- You see any blood clots.
- You are still passing large bits of scab after the first few days following the operation.

BLADDER CONTROL

The great majority of prostatectomies are successful, and recovery is usually straightforward. Having said that, though, recovery can sometimes be slow, and efficient urination is something you may have to work at.

Just after the operation, the urethra may be swollen, which may in turn be painful. This pain can make the urethral muscles contract from time to time, which can mean that the flow of urine is either slow or intermittent. Bruising of the tissues around the urethra can also prevent the muscles surrounding the urethra working properly, which can mean that the urethra neither opens nor closes completely. This can result in a low stream of urine, of continual leakage of urine. Such problems are, of course, unpleasant and debilitating, but they should disappear as soon as the swelling and bruising get better, which should take only a fortnight or so.

Another problem following the operation may be that you suffer from just as bad – if not worse – a degree of frequency and urgency of urination as you did before the operation. This is likely to be brought about by inflammation of the prostate and urethra, and may continue until the cut surface of the prostate is completely healed, which can take as long as six to eight weeks. It can last even longer if you develop a urinary tract infection, which is a good reason to have your urine tested at your six-week check-up.

It may surprise you to know that the opposite problem of an absence of urgency can, contrary to what you might expect, be even more worrying than its presence. This is because if you suffered from chronic retention of urine before your operation, your bladder may have become so accustomed to holding a large amount of urine that it does not send the right signal when it is full. The danger, in this case, is that the bladder may become so full that it will be unable to contract properly and empty itself efficiently. You will have to empty it by the clock – say every hour or so – until you begin to feel the natural urge to urinate. This should happen spontaneously, if gradually.

In short, you can expect your bladder to behaving abnormally for up to six weeks or so after the operation.

Bladder training

You will probably benefit from training – or retraining – your bladder to hold more urine and to last comfortably for longer periods of time. This should help reduce increased frequency and urgency of urination, as well as night-time urination.

Start by making a urination chart, or frequency/volume chart, detailing the time and amount of urine each time you go to the toilet. Equip yourself with a measuring jug, of the type you can buy in hardware or kitchen equipment shops, so as to measure the volume of urine. Continue keeping this chart while you are bladder training.

You will probably be used to emptying your bladder each time you feel the slightest urge to do so, or even each time you pass a toilet 'just in case'. Stop doing this and gradually increase the time between visits to the toilet. Start by holding on for another two minutes after you feel the need to go to the toilet, then increase this to five minutes, then another five minutes, and so on.

All this is easier said than done, but there are a few 'tricks' that should make it easier for you to hold on between visits.

• Sit rather than stand when you feel the desire to urinate.

• Keep still rather than moving around.

- Pull up your pelvic floor muscles (see below).
- Cross your legs.
- Hold your penis, if you can do this discreetly.
- Take regular, slow, deep breaths.
- Think about something else to keep your mind off your bladder.
- Try to do something else to take your mind off your bladder, such as making a telephone call, or reading the newspaper.

You will find that you can gradually manage to hold on for longer and longer intervals. Aim, ultimately, for an interval of three to four hours.

Bladder training can achieve a lot for most people in just four weeks. Try to keep it up for three months or, even better, six months. Don't expect to have dealt with all your problems even after six months. Symptoms can continue to improve for as long as a year – or even longer.

PELVIC FLOOR EXERCISES

Most women are familiar with their pelvic floor muscles, particularly if they have had a baby. A lot of men, on the other hand, may not even know that they have any pelvic floor muscles, let alone what or where they are.

Pelvic floor exercises strengthen the pelvic floor muscles, which support and help to close the urethra. Strengthening these muscles will help increase your ability to hold on before you go to the toilet.

Try tensing up the muscles between your scrotum and anus, in much the same way as you would to prevent the flow of urine, or to hold back the urge to break wind. If you are not sure if you are doing this right, put a finger there and you will feel a ring of muscle around the anus become firmer. Another way of doing it is to try stopping the flow of urine while you are actually urinating. If the muscles are very weak, you may only be able to weaken the flow of urine and not actually to stop it. Try this once a day until you can stop the stream of urine efficiently and completely. When you are able to tense up the muscles, you can continue practising in other positions and while doing other things – on the bus, doing the washing-up, waiting for a bus, whatever is most convenient. Hold the muscles tense for five seconds, then relax for five seconds. Repeat the whole cycle of tensing and relaxing five times, which will take about a minute. Ideally, you should do this for a total of 15 minutes (at least) a day.

You have to stick at it to obtain results, because it takes time for weakened muscles to build up strength. Stick to between three and six months of diligent exercise, and you are bound to notice results.

RESUMING SEXUAL ACTIVITY

You can resume sexual activity as soon as you feel up to it. Some doctors are wary of advising patients to do this, in case of disturbing clots and scabs, others say that the passage of semen cannot do any more harm than the passage of urine. Be alert to how you feel, and follow your natural inclinations.

You may, however, not feel like sex for some time after the operation. If this happens to you, you shouldn't worry about. It does not mean that you have lost your sex drive or your potency as a result of the operation – it simply means that you have a natural degree of fatigue after what is, after all, a major operation. This is even more likely if you have had a general anaesthetic.

Retrograde ejaculation

You are unlikely to ejaculate in quite the same way as you did before the operation and may experience retrograde ejaculation (see Chapter 7). This means that semen goes backwards up the urethra into the bladder, rather than forwards and down into the urethra. This often has the effect of making you sterile, and a lot of men find this a very difficult hurdle to deal with, even if they do not actually want to father any more children. In their eyes, the fact that they are now sterile seems to emasculate them in some way, to make them less of a man. It is important that a man is told that this is a likely side-effect of a prostatectomy before the operation, as this seems to help them deal with it better. If a man is not told until afterwards, when it is a *fait accompli* in which he had no say, he may be very angry.

Even if you do have retrograde ejaculation, this cannot guarantee that your partner won't become pregnant and you should still use some form of contraception if this is an issue. You cannot rely on a prostatectomy to give you a reliable form of contraception. It is estimated that between 5 and 10 per cent of men are still fertile afterwards. If you want a reliable and permanent method of contraception, you may want to discuss the possibility of having a vasectomy with your surgeon, as this can easily be done at the same time as a prostatectomy.

Your urine will probably look a little cloudy after intercourse, as the semen that went into the bladder is washed out. You may also find that you bleed slightly after intercourse during the first six weeks or so after the operation – just as you notice a little blood in your urine – but as long as this is not a large amount of blood, you should not have anything to worry about.

YOUR SIX-WEEK CHECK-UP

By six weeks after the operation, most of your symptoms should have cleared up, though you may still be suffering from frequency and urgency of urination.

You will probably have a check-up after six weeks, which is your opportunity to discuss anything that is worrying you.

It is particularly important to have a test done on a urine sample, just to check that you are free of any urine infection. Some hospital clinics also like to repeat the urine flow test, which will indicate that the operation has been successful.

9 Alternatives to Surgery

No treatment – orthodox treatments included – can ever be guaranteed to work perfectly every time, and can sometimes either fail to cure the condition in question, or can produce side-effects. It is therefore hardly surprising that some patients want to try alternative approaches, including some of the less conventional forms of treatment. Some patients, in any case, prefer to try the complementary, or alternative, therapies before resorting to strong drugs or to surgery.

One thing that the complementary therapies have in common is that they treat the person as a whole – including the mental, emotional, spiritual and physical aspects. This approach is rather different from that of orthodox medicine, which tends to treat individual symptoms rather than the person.

If you choose to consult a complementary therapist, always make sure that he or she is fully qualified in his or her particular field. For details of how best to contact a therapist, see the Useful Addresses on page 110.

The evidence on how well complementary therapies work in the treatment of prostate disease tends to be anecdotal. It is not generally supported by conventional rigorous clinical trials, though that does not mean you should not try them.

Keep an open mind about treatment, and don't expect miracles, any more than you would with a conventional doctor. What follows is a discussion of some of the most popular and readily available complementary approaches to prostate disease.

WARNING!

If you have the symptoms of prostate disease, you must consult your doctor before seeking complementary options. You may need to undergo tests to rule out a serious condition such as prostate cancer.

ACUPUNCTURE

Acupuncture is an ancient Chinese therapy, some 3,500 years old. Its name is based on the Latin words *acus*, meaning needle, and *punctus*, meaning to prick or puncture. This becomes clear when you know that when patients have acupuncture, they are treated by having needles put into their skin.

Needles are put into the skin at particular points, known as acupuncture points, on the body. These lie along a network of invisible energy channels, called 'meridians'. It is believed that the meridians are responsible for the flow of energy throughout the body and that they are linked to the body's internal organs. Traditional Chinese medicine is based on the belief that good health is based on a perfect balance of the energy flowing through the body.

Very fine stainless steel needles with very small heads are inserted into the acupuncture points, the idea being that they regulate the flow of energy, known as Qi, through the meridians. This may mean unblocking it, increasing it, or decreasing it – according to what is required.

Some acupuncturists also apply local heat to supplement the body's natural flow of energy. The most common way of doing this is moxibustion, which is done by placing moxa – the shredded leaves of the common mugwort – over the acupuncture point. It is then set alight and when it becomes too hot, it is removed. This may be repeated a number of times, and an acupuncture needle is then inserted as usual.

Does it work?

Acupuncture has been used in Britain since the early nineteenth century, primarily for the relief of pain and the treatment of fever, but also to stimulate the body's own ability to heal itself. It used to be dismissed as nonsense by sceptics, but the fact that it has enormous success can no longer be denied.

Acupuncturists claim success in relieving symptoms from prostate problems by using pressure points governing the bladder, large intestine, spleen and kidney. These are points on the lower abdomen and on the inner side of the lower leg.

ACUPRESSURE

Acupressure is an ancient Japanese form of therapy. It uses the same energy channels, or meridians, as acupuncture. The difference is that, instead of using needles, acupressure uses finger pressure.

If you think about it, we all use some form of acupressure – when we press our hands against our forehead when we have a headache, or when we rub a sore part of the body. The idea is that it not only brings pain relief but that it also stimulates the body's healing capacity.

As with acupuncture, a qualified practitioner in acupressure knows exactly which points to press in order to influence the prostate gland.

Does it work?

There are too many sufferers who can testify to the benefits of acupressure for its efficacy to be doubted.

REFLEXOLOGY

Reflexology is a method of treatment whereby reflex points in the feet are massaged in a particular way. The aim is to cause an effect in other parts of the body, which may well be in an altogether different area from the feet.

It has similarities to acupuncture and acupressure in that it is based on the same principle – namely that energy flows through the body along invisible energy channels, or meridians. The difference in this case is that the terminal points of the meridians are in the feet.

Reflexology dates back some 5,000 years to China and, subsequently, to ancient Egypt. In more recent times, there is evidence that reflexology has been used by some of the Red Indian tribes and by the primitive tribes of Africa.

The first modern-day use of reflexology, also known as zone therapy, can be attributed to Dr William H. Fitzgerald, who worked as an ear, nose and throat specialist in America at the beginning of this century. He developed his theory of reflexology and mapped out the meridians of the body, ending in the feet and hands. Using the thumbs and fingers, the reflexologist will balance the body's flow of energy by stimulating various terminal points in the feet.

Does it work?

All the reproductive gland disorders, both female and male – of which the prostate gland is one – respond particularly well to reflexology. As with all the complementary therapies, it is particularly important to consult a fully qualified therapist.

HERBAL TREATMENT

Herbalism has been around for a long time. It was, in fact, the most common form of medical treatment in the West right up until the eighteenth century.

The use of herbs as a method of treatment has retained much of its popularity throughout the world to this day. Herbalists say that herbs enhance the body's natural healing powers.

Caution is advised when using herbal remedies. Many herbs can be highly beneficial, but they must be used in carefully controlled doses. This means that they must be prescribed by someone who knows what they are doing. The random use of herbs or incorrect handling can, in fact, be dangerous, which is why it is so important to consult a qualified herbalist and not to self-medicate.

Does it work?

Herbalists claim success with most kinds of illness, though it should be realised that herbalism is often slower to have an effect than conventional medicine.

A non-cancerous enlarged prostate often responds to herbal teas. Non-cancerous prostate enlargement and associated difficulty in passing water respond particularly well to a number of diuretic herbs, such as couch grass, horsetail or saw palmetto, to provoke the release of urine. A good healing diuretic can be made in an infusion of 10g each of dried white deadnettle, cornsilk and pellitory-of-the-wall; take this two or three times a day.

If the problem is one of increased frequency of urination and associated discomfort, a decoction of equal quantities of gravel root, sea holly and hydrangea root taken at a dosage of 45-60 ml/3-4 tablespoonfuls three times a day will reduce inflammation and thereby help ease the problem.

Other herbs that are thought to ease prostate problems include club moss, damiana, horse chestnut, golden rod, greater celandine, ladies' mantle, mallow, nettles, parsley, rosemary, St John's wort, white deadnettle, wild thyme, and the small-flowered willow herb.

HOMOEOPATHY

Homoeopathy has been around for nearly 200 years, when a German doctor called Samuel Hahnemann developed a new system of treatment as an alternative to the conventional form of medicine that was being practised at the time. Conventional medical practices included such procedures as blood-letting and purging, which Hahnemann considered to be too severe and to tend to weaken patients rather than to heal them. Hahnemann's aim was to come up with a new system based on gentle ways of helping the body to heal itself.

It was Hahnemann's belief that a person's symptoms are a sign that he or she is trying to resist illness. "Far from seeking a way to suppress symptoms, it may be desirable to take some form of treatment calculated to help the resistance."

A breakthrough came when Hahnemann discovered that if a healthy person took a herbal remedy for malaria, cinchona tree bark, it actually provoked symptoms of the disease, such as headache and a high temperature. This discovery in fact revived an ancient principle, first formulated by the Greek physician Hippocrates in the fifth century B.C., that 'like cures like'. Hahnemann believed that small doses were actually more effective than big ones, and devised a system – still little understood by many doctors to this day, of diluting doses to the maximum degree.

Hahnemann called his new system of medicine homoeopathy, from the Greek words 'homoios', meaning like, and 'pathos', meaning suffering. It is a complex system, whose aim is to restore the body's natural balance and to strengthen its resistance to disease.

He spent years trying out his beliefs not only on himself but also on his family and friends. He used a wide range of natural substances and developed an extensive homoeopathic pharmacopoeia.

Does it work?

Clinical trials on homoeopathy have had mixed results: some have claimed success, others have shown no significant improvement.

In spite of this, however, many homoeopaths claim that their remedies are actually much more effective than conventional medicine, and there are many patients who have been successfully treated and who would agree with this.

There are literally hundreds of possible homoeopathic remedies from the plant and animal world that are beneficial to men suffering from prostate problems. Prescribing the right remedy for your particular problem is not a simple matter of do-it-yourself but must be put in the hands of a qualified homoeopath, who will select a remedy with reference to the patient's personality rather than just the patient's prostate.

NATUROPATHY

We may not realise it but we all practise naturopathic treatment from time to time. Every time you bathe a sore part of the body, stop eating when your stomach is upset, or sweat out a fever, you are practising naturopathy.

Naturopathy aims to help the body to cure itself in a number of ways. These include dietary measures, exercise and water treatment.

Does it work?

Naturopathy has a large and pleasing measure of common sense about it.

Naturopathic procedures recommended for prostate problems include hot and cold compresses. Also recommended are hot and cold sitz baths, which are the partial immersion in a bath of the pelvic region. They are more easily given in a specially constructed bath, but may also be performed in an ordinary bath-tub. Another form of hydrotherapy, or water treatment, is to sit in hot water with the feet in cold water for 3 minutes, and then change over to sitting in cold water with the feet in hot water for 1 minute.

Dietary recommendations are to maintain a wholefood diet, preferably an organic diet with as little exposure as possible to pesticides and other environmental contaminants. Avoid refined carbohydrates, coffee, strong tea and alcohol, particularly beer. If you are suffering from an enlarged prostate, increase your intake of zinc-rich foods, such as pumpkin seeds (about 25g/1 oz seeds a day). Alternatively, there are a number of recommended supplements that have been found to be effective in the treatment of an enlarged prostate. Some of these are widely used in Continental Europe, where they are often prescribed to men who are being treated for an enlarged prostate. Many of the men treated in this way report a dramatic improvement in symptoms, particularly with extracts of rye pollen (see below).

Natural treatments include a number of preparations. These are:

- Extracts of rye pollen, such as Cernilton and ProstaBrit. Rye pollen has been used to treat an enlarged prostate in Continental Europe since the 1960s, and has been shown to be effective in several clinical trials. There are very few reported side-effects, mild heartburn and nausea being the most common ones.

- Golden rod *(Solidago)*, which is widely used in Continental Europe, where it is claimed to be responsible for a dramatic improvement in symptoms.

- South African stargrass, such as Harzol, also used in Continental Europe. This has not as yet been subjected to clinical trials.

- African prune *(Pygeum africanum)*, such as Tadenan, also used in Continental Europe.

- American dwarf saw palmetto *(Serenoa repens)*. This is a small palm tree native to the Atlantic coast of North America from south Carolina to Florida, growing up to 10 feet high with a crown of large leaves. The dark red/brown berries of the palm were used by the American Indians and later by naturopaths and homoeopaths to treat genito-urinary tract disorders. Extract of the berries, such as Permixon, have been shown in clinical studies to improve prostate enlargement, due to the inhibition of dihydrotestosterone. Take 160 mg twice daily.

- Zinc, which digital rectal examinations have shown to reduce the size of the prostate gland. The best supplemental form of zinc to use is probably zinc picolinate, and the recommended dose is 60 mg a day for a maximum of six months. The absorption of zinc is reduced by alcohol.

- Vitamin B6 (pyridoxine), which increases the absorption of zinc. Take 100-125 mg per day. Again, alcohol is known to reduce the absorption of vitamin B6 levels.

- Essential fatty acids, the administration of which has been shown to result in significant improvement for many sufferers of prostate enlargement. One teaspoonful or 4 g of oil twice daily is recommended, or 3-6 capsules a day. Linseed oil, sunflower oil, evening primrose oil, walnut oil and soya oil are all appropriate oils to add to the diet.

- Ginseng, which is one of the most widely used plants in Oriental medicine and has a long historical folk use in prostate enlargement, though no clinical trials have been done. Take 2-4 g of the dried root three times daily, or 25-50 mg extract daily.

- kombucha, which is a tea fermented from the kombucha plant indigenous to Eastern Europe. This works by refining the body's metabolism and boosting the immune system. In Eastern Europe, the kombucha tonic is believed to have the magical ability to delay ageing. It has been found to be especially effective in treating prostate problems and, in particular, in combating impotence. Drink two or three cups of kombucha tea a day.

- Royal jelly, which is manufactured in the beehive for the sole consumption of the queen bee and has been found to relieve symptoms of a diseased prostate in humans, particularly a sense of burning on urination. Take two capsules of royal jelly three times a day.

10 Living with your Prostate

We hope we have shown you two things: firstly, you need to be aware of your prostate gland and what can go wrong with it, so that you can get treatment for any possible problems if they arise; and secondly, even if problems do arise, they are unlikely to be as bad as you may fear, and can probably be completely cured.

BE AWARE AND DON'T DESPAIR are the key words when it comes to the prostate.

A positive outlook on life is one of the greatest weapons we have at our disposal.

Never forget it.

BE AWARE

It is important to keep an eye on any changes in your urinary habits, particularly after the age of 50. Changes may creep up on you slowly over the years, but don't use that as an excuse for not taking them seriously.

Ask yourself the following questions:

- Do you have to get up at night to urinate?
- Do you urinate much more often than you used to?
- Do you have difficulty passing water?
- Is your flow of urine particularly thin or weak, particularly in the morning?
- Do you ever experience any pain when you urinate?

- Do you ever notice any blood in your urine?
- Can you urinate as high, or as far, as you used to?
- Do you get pains in the region of your prostate, in the groin, or around your genitals?
- Do you sometimes find it difficult to start the flow of urine?
- Do you sometimes find that you involuntarily stop and start urinating?
- Do you sometimes feel as though you haven't quite emptied your bladder and there's more to come?
- Do you have to strain to pass water?
- Do you ever suffer from incontinence?
- Does your urine continue dribbling, even when you think you've finished?
- Do you sometimes need to rush urgently to the toilet to urinate?
- Do you ever notice blood in your semen?

Warning symptoms

If you have answered Yes to one (or more) of these questions, you may be experiencing problems with your prostate. Warning signs of this kind are there to be taken notice of, and you should never ignore them.

Men are notoriously good at sweeping under the carpet things that make them feel uncomfortable, and signs that all may not be quite as they should be on the health front come into this category. The reason why you should not do this is a straightforward, not to say obvious, one. It is, quite simply, because the sooner you do something about them, the greater your chances of doing something constructive about them and effecting a cure.

Men also tend to be frightened of wasting their doctor's time and being viewed as a nuisance. But you shouldn't worry about this, your doctor is very unlikely to think this way. Doctors are there to look after your health, and if something is really worrying you that's enough to warrant a visit.

So the message is:

GO TO SEE YOUR DOCTOR.

CONSULTING YOUR DOCTOR

First of all, your doctor will want to know all your symptoms. To make sure you don't forget to tell him about any of these, make a list of them before you go to the surgery. You should also make a note of any questions you want to ask him.

The doctor will take a general medical history, with particular reference to any serious familial diseases such as diabetes, heart disease or haemophilia, and any drugs you are taking. He will also want to know about any important changes in your health that you have noticed recently, such as general fatigue or lower back pain, which may not seem to you to be at all relevant but which could be important to the doctor.

If you're worried about your urinary habits, it's as well to establish a relationship with your doctor, so you can get to know him and he can get to know you and your anxieties. If you're just starting to have symptoms, he may not find anything much wrong now, but he will want you both to keep an eye on things and to monitor the situation.

Above all, never be embarrassed to talk to your doctor about your urinary habits. He won't be embarrassed and you shouldn't be either.

YOUR LIFESTYLE

There are several changes you can make to your lifestyle which will help keep your prostate healthy.

Try to do the following:

- Don't smoke. Smoking causes spasm in smooth muscle and

may, as a result, make matters worse, particularly if a prostate problem has already been diagnosed.

- Keep your consumption of alcohol, which can irritate the bladder, as low as possible. In particular, avoid beer.
- Avoid coffee. Coffee has an irritating effect on the bladder at the best of times, and if the bladder is already 'unstable', this effect is likely to be heightened.
- Try to keep stress in your life to a minimum, as it can intensify urinary problems such as hesitancy and urgency. This is easier said than done, but you may benefit (wouldn't we all?) from making every effort not to allow yourself to be too easily worked up by the pressures of modern-day life. Try learning some relaxation techniques.
- Try to avoid going out in the cold, which can often trigger bladder problems.
- Wrap up warm.
- Get plenty of sleep.
- Take regular exercise. In particular, it is thought that having played a lot of sport regularly as a child, particularly before reaching puberty, may have a protective effect against the development of cancer of the prostate. Exercise is still beneficial in adult life because it keeps the muscles around the abdomen active.
- Don't regularly restrict your fluid intake because you are frightened of having to go to the loo too often. Drinking less may not actually help anyway. If you have an important meeting, or are going to the theatre, restrict your fluid intake from about three hours beforehand, which should help make it easier for you to go out. You can also restrict fluid intake at night, which may mean you don't have to get up so often to urinate.

DIET

The main thing you can do to protect your prostate and to

prevent it from causing you problems later in life is to follow a prostate-friendly diet.

The idea of a diet that's good for the heart has been around for a long time and people are slowly becoming better educated about this and following the advice given. But a diet that's good for the prostate is a relatively new idea and not something that most men take very seriously.

But before you dismiss this idea as being silly or unnecessary, remember, prostate disease is terribly common. The more you can do about keeping it at bay, the better.

Dietary tips

- Keep your intake of saturated fats (butter, animal fats, palm oil, coconut oil) to a minimum, as the latest research shows that it can increase the risk of prostate cancer.

- Switch to low-fat milk, cheese, dressings, etc.

- Reduce your consumption of meat, in particular red meat, which you should eat either not at all or only occasionally.

- Remove the skin from chicken.

- Increase your consumption of fish. Fish oil may have anti-cancer benefits.

- Eat a diet that is rich in fibre (fruit and vegetables, particularly potatoes and sweetcorn), wholemeal bread, pulses, brown rice and pasta. Fibre reduces the chances of constipation, and regular constipation can put pressure on the prostate gland.

- Try to eat a minimum of five portions of fruit or vegetables each day. Ideally, eat them raw or only lightly cooked.

- Drink plenty of fluids – around 1.75-2.25 litres/3-4 pints a day – as this also helps prevent constipation. Drink milk, mineral waters and diluted fruit juices rather than alcohol or coffee, both of which are diuretics. Drinking sufficient fluids also helps protect your bladder from infections.

- Eat plenty of nuts and seeds. The World Health Organization (WHO) recommend that everyone should eat at least 30 g of nuts or seeds per day.

- Green, yellow and orange fruits and vegetables are particularly beneficial because they are rich in beta-carotene, which converts to vitamin A in the intestine and liver, and has an antioxidant effect which is thought to protect against cancer. Rich sources of beta-carotene include carrots, oranges and apricots.

- Make sure your diet is rich in vitamins C and E, because of their ability to mop up dangerous free radicals which can form during the body's metabolic processes and thus weaken their protective powers against cancer. Foods rich in vitamin C include most fruits and vegetables, particularly citrus fruits, strawberries, potatoes and peppers; while foods rich in vitamin E include most vegetable oils, eggs, fish, green leafy vegetables and pulses.

- Make sure your diet is rich in zinc. Good sources of zinc include shellfish (particularly oysters), fish (particularly herrings), wholegrain cereals, oatmeal, eggs, cheese, nuts and seeds (particularly pumpkin and sunflower seeds).

- Make sure your diet is rich in essential fatty acids, such as sunflower oil, safflower oil, linseed oil, walnut oil and soya oil.

- You may find that spicy foods have an adverse effect on your prostate problems. This is because they upset the bowel, and the prostate rests against it.

- You may find it helpful to keep a diary of the food you eat and your symptoms; this should help you work out what foods or drinks precipitate symptoms, and you can then avoid them.

Food supplements

- Take zinc supplements (around 10 mg three times a day). If this amount upsets your stomach or makes you feel nauseous, both of which are possible side-effects, you can reduce your dose (10 mg just twice a day).

- Take evening primrose oil.

- If you're worried about your diet, take dietary supplements. Take vitamin C (around 150 mg a day); vitamin E (around 30-40 mg a day); and beta-carotene (around 15 mg a day). These are all antioxidants and can help reduce inflammation as well as protecting against cancer.

Your Questions Answered

Q. I was due to have surgery for an enlarged prostate in a few weeks, but I had a heart attack two months ago. My doctor says that I should leave a gap of at least three months after my heart attack before I have surgery for my prostate. I am reluctant to wait because the symptoms are quite severe and they are really getting me down. Is my doctor right?

A. Yes, he is. It would be unwise for surgery to take place within three months of a heart attack, as the risks of another attack are too high. Some people might actually suggest that you wait six months, by which time the risks will have fallen dramatically. An enlarged prostate can be very irritating but it is not a matter of life or death, a heart attack is, so be patient and wait until you are fit enough to undergo surgery. You might also like to talk to your specialist about the possibility of having surgery under a spinal anaesthetic rather than a general one.

Q. Why might a repeat prostate operation become necessary?

A. A repeat operation may become necessary because of regrowth of obstructing prostate tissue. Obviously, the younger a man is when he has his first prostate operation, the more likely he is to need a repeat operation later on. Similarly, the longer he lives, the greater his chance of needing a second operation. About 15 per cent of patients need to have a repeat operation within 15 years.

Q. My father and my grandfather both had cancer of the prostate. I have heard that this makes it much more likely that I will develop this disease too. Is this true, and is there anything I can do to prevent it? I am 32 years old.

A. It is true that men who have a family history of prostate cancer have a higher risk of developing the same disease. This does not mean, however, that it is by any means inevitable, and you should not look on the black side.

You are right, though, to be alerted to the possible problem. You should, of course, lead as healthy a life as you can, following a healthy diet, not drinking alcohol excessively, not smoking, minimising stress and getting plenty of exercise.

Other than that, you may be able to persuade your doctor to refer you for regular screening because of your family's medical history. Although men are unlikely to develop prostate cancer until they are over 50 years old, it would be wise to start a screening programme now and repeat tests every five years. This should reassure you.

Q. Is it true that prostate surgery always causes a man to become impotent?

A. No, this is absolutely not true. It used to be truer in the past than it is today. It is the nerves that run on either side of the prostate that control a man's ability to obtain and maintain an erection. The techniques used in prostate surgery nowadays do not usually disturb these nerves. A small minority of patients do, however, suffer some degree of impotence, though no one is quite sure why this should be. It has been suggested that the causes may sometimes be psychological rather than physical, though this is not always the case.

Q. I have been diagnosed as having an enlarged prostate, which I understand is benign. Is there any danger that this might turn into prostate cancer if I do not have it removed?

A. No, there is no link between an enlarged prostate and prostate cancer. The exact cause of an enlarged prostate is not fully understood, and neither is the cause of prostate cancer, but the two are not connected. It is true that prostate cancer is occasionally diagnosed when a man is being operated on for an enlarged prostate, but the link here is only one of diagnosis, not cause. It is one of the hidden benefits of prostate surgery, in fact, that if there is any cancer of the prostate that has not been discovered already, it will be found when the prostate is operated on.

Q. Are there any easy remedies that one can buy at the chemists and which will cure prostate enlargement?

A. No. There are some that may reduce symptoms, but this is not the same as a cure. Anyone who makes claims to the contrary is being economical with the truth.

Q. I'm thinking of having a vasectomy. I've heard that a vasectomy can cause cancer of the prostate. Is this true?

A. A link has been suggested but it is most unlikely. There is no definitely proven link between vasectomy and prostate cancer, but if this is something that particularly worries you, you should obviously discuss this with your consultant.

Q. My girlfriend tells me that she has had chlamydia. This • happened when she was younger and before she met me. I have heard that chlamydia can be linked with a prostate problem, called prostatitis. Is she putting me at risk?

A. It is true that prostatitis is thought to be linked sometimes • with chlamydia. But if your girlfriend had chlamydia before she met you and is now completely clear of it, it doesn't sound as though you have anything to worry about. If you want to be completely on the safe side, though, why don't you both go to your local genito-urinary medicine (GUM) clinic (you'll find the number in your telephone directory) and ask for a check-up. Explain what it is that's worrying you and they will be happy to help. You do not need to feel at all embarrassed about going to a genito-urinary clinic, the staff are always very sympathetic, friendly and matter-of-fact about these matters, and will do everything they can to make you feel at home. Don't worry, either, that they'll think you're wasting their time. So often, problems are caused by people who really ought to go to the clinic and, for whatever reason, don't go until it's too late, either to treat their disease easily, or to prevent them from passing it on to other people. They will be delighted that you have made a move before it becomes a problem.

Q. My father died recently from a stroke. His doctor told me • that he had prostate cancer, but that his was a silent disease. What does this mean, and did this have anything to do with his death?

A. It means that his cancer was not spreading and was not • causing him any great problem. It was certainly not that which killed him. You do not say how old your father was, but prostate cancer of this sort is very common in elderly men. It is often never even diagnosed and only comes to light during a post-mortem. Even when it is diagnosed, it often does not require any treatment, precisely because it is a silent disease.

Q. I have had chronic bacterial prostatitis for some years now. Although recurrences are not as regular as they used to be, I do still have occasional flare-ups. My wife has been trying to get pregnant – with no success – for about a year. Is there any connection and, if so, what are our chances?

A. There is some indication that certain forms of prostatitis, particularly chronic bacterial prostatitis, may result in lower male fertility. Infection or inflammation of the prostate can cause certain changes in the prostatic fluid, which may well affect the quality of the semen, and therefore a man's fertility. Your best bet would be to discuss this with your doctor and to have both your sperm count and sperm quality checked. This is a simple test which is done from a sample of semen following ejaculation by masturbation.

Useful Addresses

Better Prostate Healthline
Tel: 0891 667788

British Association of Cancer United Patients (BACUP)
3 Bath Place
Rivington Street
London EC2A 3JR
Tel: 0800 181199
10.00 a.m.-7.00 p.m. Monday to Thursday;
10.00 a.m.-5.30 p.m. Friday.

Human Fertilisation and Embryology Authority
Paxton House
30 Artillery Lane
London E1 7LS
Tel: 0171-377 5077

British Pregnancy Advisory Service
Austy Manor
Wootton Wawen
Solihull
West Midlands B95 6BX
Tel: 0121-643 1461

Cancer Aid and Listening Line (CALL)
Swan Buildings
20 Swan Street
Manchester M4 5VW
Tel: 0161-434 8668

Cancer Support Centre
PO Box 17
20-22 York Road
London SW11 3QE
Tel: 0171-924 3924

CancerLink
17 Britannia Street
London WC1X 9JN
Tel: 0171-833 2451

Marie Stopes
153/157 Cleveland Street
London W1P 5PG
Tel: 0171-574 7400

ProstaBrit Information Service
Greatness Lane
Sevenoaks
Kent TN14 5BQ
Tel: 01737-773304

Prostate Help Association
Langworth
Lincoln LN3 5DF
No telephone support.

THE COMPLEMENTARY OPTIONS (see Chapter 9)

ACUPUNCTURE
British Acupuncture Association and Register
34 Alderney Street
London SW1V 4EU
Tel: 0171-834 1012

Council for Acupuncture
Park House
206 Latimer Road
London W10 6RE
Tel: 0181-964 0222

HERBALISM
The National Institute of Medical Herbalists
56 Longbrook Street
Exeter EX4 6AH
Tel: 01392-426022

HOMOEOPATHY
The British Homoeopathic Association
27a Devonshire Street
London W1N 1RJ
Tel: 0171-935 2163

The Homoeopathic Society
(formerly Hahnemann Society)
2 Powis Place
Great Ormond Street
London WC1N 3HT
Tel: 0171-837 9469

The Homoeopathic Trust
2 Powis Place
Great Ormond Street
London WC1N 3HT
Tel: 0171-837 9469

NATUROPATHY

The British Naturopathic Association
Goswell House
2 Goswell Road
Street
Somerset BA16 0JG
Tel: 01458-840072

REFLEXOLOGY

Association of Reflexologists
27 Old Gloucester Street
London WC1N 3XX
Tel: 01892-512612

Glossary

ACUTE – Often used to describe a disorder, or symptom, that comes on suddenly. An acute condition may or may not be severe, but it is usually of short duration.

ANDROGENS – Bodily hormones that help in the development of male sex characteristics. Testosterone is the most important of these.

ANUS – The exterior opening, through which waste products are excreted, located at the end of the digestive tract.

BACTERIA – A group of single-celled micro-organisms, many – though not all – of which cause diseases.

BENIGN – Not malignant. Characteristic of a mild illness. Recovery is likely.

BIOPSY – The removal of tissue from a patient so that it may be studied under a microscope in order to make a precise diagnosis.

BLADDER – An elastic sac that stores urine before it is excreted from the body.

BOGGY – A term used to describe the prostate when it is swollen, spongy and soft.

CANCER – A group of diseases in which symptoms are due to the uncontrolled growth of abnormal cells creating a cellular tumour. These cells can spread throughout the body through the bloodstream or the lymphatic system.

CAPSULE – The structure in which an item, such as the prostate, is enclosed.

CATHETER – A hollow, flexible, surgical tube that is used to drain or inject fluid. It is used, in particular, to drain urine via the urethra from the bladder.

CAT SCAN (CT SCAN) – A diagnostic imaging technique using X-rays and computer technology to provide cross-sectional pictures of the body.

CHLAMYDIA – A group of non-bacterial infections in the urethra and genital tract, and one of the most common sexually-transmitted diseases.

CHRONIC – A chronic condition is one that persists for a long time (sometimes in spite of treatment).

CYSTOSCOPE – A lighted viewing instrument that is inserted up the urethra in order to examine the urethra and the bladder.

DYSURIA – Pain on passing urine.

EJACULATION – The act of emission of semen from the penis.

ENZYME – A protein that regulates the rate of a chemical reaction in the body. Every cell in the body produces various enzymes.

ERECTION – The stiffening, hardening and elevation that occur in the penis in response to sexual arousal.

FREQUENCY – The need to urinate at short intervals.

GENITALS – The reproductive organs – both male and female, both internal and external.

GENITO-URINARY – Referring to a man's or woman's reproductive and urinary tract.

GLAND – A group of specialised cells that manufacture and release certain chemicals, including hormones and enzymes, for use in the body.

HAEMATURIA – Blood in the urine.

HAEMOSPERMIA – Blood in the seminal fluid.

HESITANCY – Slowness to start the initial urinary flow.

HORMONE – A chemical that is released into the bloodstream by a particular gland or tissue and which has a specific effect on tissues elsewhere in the body.

HYPERPLASIA – Cell proliferation.

HYPERTROPHY – The excessive, abnormal growth of an organ.

IMPOTENCE – Inability to achieve a good enough erection for sexual intercourse.

INCONTINENCE, URINARY – Inability to control the passing of urine.

INTERMITTENCY – Stopping and starting the flow of urine, often resulting in an inability to empty the bladder completely.

INTRAVENOUS PYELOGRAM (IVP) – Also known as urography. A diagnostic procedure for taking X-ray pictures of the urinary tract. A dye – or, to give its proper name, a radio-opaque medium – is injected intravenously into the bloodstream, which then shows up on X-rays when it is excreted by the kidneys, ureter and bladder.

KIDNEYS – Two small organs located on either side of the spinal column. Impurities in the blood are removed in the kidneys and dissolved to form urine.

LASER – An acronym, which stands for Light Amplification by Stimulated Emission of Radiation. Laser beams, which are concentrations of light and heat, can be used to cut, and are now being employed increasingly in surgery.

LIBIDO – Sexual desire.

MALIGNANT – Not benign. Cancerous, with the ability to invade other tissues, and to spread, or metastasise, throughout the body.

METASTASIS – A resulting cancer that has spread from another part of the body. Metastases are spread by the bloodstream or the lymph system.

MID-STREAM URINE (MSU) – A urine sample is taken mid-way in the flow of urination – neither at the beginning nor at the end, which gives less opportunity for contamination from surrounding tissues. This gives the best sample for culture or analysis.

NOCTURIA – The urge to urinate during the night, which wakes you up and means you have to get up to go to the toilet. Normally, the kidneys will produce less urine during the night when you are asleep, and the bladder will not signal that it is full until the morning. If the bladder is irritable, however, or if there is residual urine left over in the bladder, a man will be woken by the sensation of a full bladder.

ORCHIDECTOMY – The surgical removal of one or both testicles.

ORGASM – The ultimate climax of the sexual act. In a man, ejaculation normally occurs at this point.

PEAK URINE FLOW – The maximum urine flow that a man can produce, measured in millilitres per second.

PERINEUM – The area between the scrotum and anus.

PROSTATECTOMY – The surgical removal of all or part of the prostate gland.

PROSTATE GLAND – Male gland, about the size of a chestnut, through which the urethra, or urinary pipe, passes.

RADIATION – Energy that is emitted in the form of waves or particles of light. Used in medicine for both diagnosis and treatment.

RADIOTHERAPY – The use of radiation in medicine for the treatment of disease, usually cancer.

RESECTOSCOPE – A surgical instrument that allows the surgeon to see inside the urethra and is used in a transurethral prostatectomy (TURP).

SCROTUM – The pouch at a man's crotch containing the testicles.

SEMEN – The fluid that is produced by the male on ejaculation.

SEMINAL FLUID - The fluid that is emitted by the penis when a man ejaculates.

SECRETIONS - The manufacture and release by a gland, cell or organ of chemical substances.

SEXUALLY-TRANSMITTED DISEASE - One of the many diseases that can be transmitted through sexual relations. Used to be known as venereal disease.

SITZ BATH - A sit-down bath, which can be beneficial to people suffering from rectal and urinary problems.

SPERM - The male sex cell produced by the testes, also known as spermatozoon (singular) or spermatozoa (plural), which can fertilise the female egg, or ovum.

STERILITY - The inability of a man to father children.

TESTICLES - A man's two reproductive glands located in his scrotum. The testicles produce sperm and androgens (primarily testosterone).

ULTRASOUND - Also known as sonography. A diagnostic technique in which very high frequency sound waves are passed into the body, and reflected echoes are analysed to build up a picture of the internal organs. The procedure is entirely safe, and quite painless.

URETHRA - Urinary pipe which passes through the penis, through which urine passes from the bladder to the outside. Seminal fluids also pass through the urethra during ejaculation.

URINARY FLOW RATE – How quickly urine is voided from the bladder at the peak of urination. If the urinary flow is weaker than normal, it may indicate that there is some urethral obstruction.

URINE – The pale yellow fluid produced by the kidneys, which is excreted fom the body via the bladder and the urethra.

URINE CULTURE – The study of a sample of urine to allow the growth of micro-organisms. This allows a urinary tract infection to be identified.

UROLOGIST – Doctor specialising in disorders of the urinary tract and the male genital tract.

VASECTOMY – Male sterilisation, performed by cutting through the vas deferens on each side of the body, which carry sperm from the testicles to the urethra.

X-RAY – Probably the best known of all imaging techniques, first discovered by Wilhelm Konrad Röntgen in 1895. It is a useful diagnostic procedure, using electromagnetic radiations of short wave length, which produce high-quality images of bones, organs and internal tissues.

Personal Prostate Record

Personal Prostate Record

Personal Prostate Record

Personal Prostate Record

Personal Prostate Record

Personal Prostate Record

Personal Prostate Record

Personal Prostate Record